Power and Compassion

The Guilford Family Therapy Series
Michael P. Nichols, *Series Editor*

Recent Volumes

POWER AND COMPASSION

Working with Difficult Adolescents and Abused Parents

JEROME A. PRICE

Foreword by Cloé Madanes

THE GUILFORD PRESS
New York   London

Last digit is print number: 9 8 7 6 5 4 3

Library of Congress Cataloging-in-Publication Data

Price, Jerome A.
    Power and compassion : working with difficult adolescents
and abused parents / Jerome A. Price
        p.   cm. — (The Guilford Family Therapy Series).
    Includes bibliographical references and index.
    ISBN 1-57230-141-4 (hard.)—1-57230-470-7 (pbk. July 1999)
    1. Aggressiveness (Psychology) in adolescence. 2. Oppositional defiant
disorder in adolescence. 3. Abused parents. I. Title. II. Series.
RJ506.A35P75   1996
616.89′022—dc20   96-29012
                                                                        CIP

Permission to reprint the following material is gratefully acknowledged:
Part of the Introduction is reprinted from *Journal of Systemic Therapies*, *12*(4), Winter,
1993. © 1993 by Jerome A. Price. Chapter 2 is adapted from *Journal of Strategic and Systemic Therapies*, *7*(4), Winter, 1988. © 1988 by Jerome A. Price. Part of Chapter 4 is
adapted from *Family Therapy Networker*, July/August, 1989; and *Utne Reader*, *42*, No-
vember/December, 1990. © 1989 and 1990 by Jerome A. Price. Chapter 7 is adapted
from *Journal of Systemic Therapies*, *13*(3), Fall, 1994. © 1994 by Jerome A. Price. Chapter 8 is adapted from *Family Therapy Networker*, July/August, 1990. © 1990 by Jerome
A. Price. Excerpts from *Ordinary People* (Guest, 1976, pp. 109–112) appear in Chapter
4. © 1976 by Judith Guest. Reprinted by permission from Viking Penguin, a division of
Penguin Books USA Inc., and HarperCollins Publishers Limited. Excerpts from *Mys-

For Jan

Foreword

Power and Compassion offers the practicing therapist an extensive range of therapeutic interventions to solve the more serious and difficult problems of adolescents—problems involving aggressive or self-destructive acts, abuse of drugs or alcohol, bizarre communication, and extreme apathy or depression.

Clinicians have always had difficulty describing the social context of the disturbing adolescent. In the decades of the 1960s and 1970s an awareness developed about the importance of family structures. It was noted that young people with symptoms live in family hierarchies that are incorrect in some way, as when there are no generation lines or when a child determines what happens in a family. The issue became how to describe problem hierarchies and how to think about changing them.

Years ago I suggested that the social organizations of problem young people have dual hierarchies which require conflicting levels of communication. The difficulties of the young person, the trouble he causes, or her failure in life become the main theme in the parents' lives. The youth might passively threaten that if he is stressed he will go crazy or take drugs or harm himself in some way, or she might physically attack the parents. The parents become unable to attempt to change the young person's behavior because they are afraid that they will cause her harm or that she will harm them. Parents and child are caught in two incongruous hierarchies that conflict paradoxically. In one, the youth is incompetent, defective, and dependent on the parents for protection, food, shelter, and money, and the parents are in a superior position and provide for and take care of him. Yet, simultaneously, another hierarchy is defined in which the parents are dominated by the youth because of his helplessness or threats or dangerous behavior. For such cases, I proposed a method of therapy using simple, straightforward techniques to empower parents.

This book takes the next step. Jerome Price suggests a new view that might appear obvious, yet goes against so much prejudice in our profession. He views parents of aggressive adolescents not just as caught in conflicting hierarchies, but as abuse victims rather than victimizers, suggesting that violent young people have not necessarily become this way as a result of any kind of mistreatment. He discusses the causes of parent abuse and describes identifiable patterns in the interactions of families where parents are victimized by their children. The power tactics used by teens to perpetrate emotional abuse on their parents are brilliantly described and counter tactics are offered.

Price has the courage and insight to go against the trend in our culture toward parent blaming and recognizes the abusive techniques and emotional terrorism used by young people to exploit and befuddle adults. In a society where parent bashing is the norm, this is a brave stance.

The book brings common sense and the voice of reason to very difficult problems. Price offers a variety of new and unusual ways to intervene to stop parental abuse and correct the disturbing behavior of young people. There are two possible pitfalls a reader should bear in mind. One is a danger common to all strategic therapy: the possibility of applying the techniques mechanically without understanding the particular situation of a family. The other is the danger that the focus on parent abuse may lead to a view of the family from one perspective only. Price is aware of both dangers and is careful to caution the reader.

This book clarifies issues of hierarchy, guilt, responsibility, and interpersonal influence that have fascinated therapists for a long time. Readers will learn not only new ways of doing therapy but also better ways of parenting their own children.

CLOÉ MADANES
Family Therapy Institute
Rockville, Maryland

Acknowledgments

I believe that very little in the field of therapy is independently developed. Whether consciously or unconsciously, we are influenced by those who came before us, spoke to us, and wrote books and articles for us to read. I therefore want to thank all of those therapists and theorists who have influenced my thinking and made this book possible.

Particularly, I'd like to thank Salvador Minuchin who, without knowing me, introduced me to and excited me about family therapy. My deepest gratitude goes to Cloé Madanes and Jay Haley for patiently teaching me how to successfully do what I'd become interested in. They are directly and indirectly responsible for many of the ideas in this book.

I want to personally acknowledge the efforts and support of those who read and reread copies of the manuscript and provided invaluable input on ideas and form—particularly, my wife, Jan, and colleagues and friends, Julie Stitt and Elizabeth Gordon. My special thanks to Thomas Blume for consulting on the accuracy of the chapter "He Must Be on Drugs," and to Reverend Suzanne Paul and Reverend Penny Hackett-Evans for providing me with resources about humanism for the introduction. Richard Schwartz was kind enough to send me material from his upcoming book which contributed to the clarity of Chapter 8. Finally, I'm indebted to my editor, Michael Nichols, who believed in *Power and Compassion*, and went above and beyond the call of duty by pushing me to make this book all it could be and by lending his vision and expertise on all aspects of its development.

Contents

Introduction

Change is a mystery that therapists explore. There are as many ways to intervene in a problem as there are therapists, and most approaches are reasonably effective. Confusion arises, though, when therapists are faced with unmanageable young people who overwhelm their parents while damaging their own lives.

Many therapists are following the pendulum of current conventional wisdom and have accepted the modern idea that these destructive situations occur because the rights of young people are being violated and their self-determination is being denied them. If we listen to the complaints of disgruntled young people, we'll hear a litany of objections to any attempt at authoritarian parenting.

Typically, systemic therapists, and particularly strategists, embrace a hierarchical approach to serious problems of adolescence. They see the need for more leadership from parents—less talk, more action. Therapists tend to be extremists by nature and therefore feel compelled to take one position regarding the cause of adolescent problems. But our clinical advantage of objectivity is lost if we as therapists allow ourselves to become caught up in one or another dichotomous position—toughness versus tenderness, more rules versus more understanding.

Just because young people who are becoming aggressive and dominating are seizing more and more power, it doesn't necessarily follow that they are this way as a result of mistreatment (even though they may indeed have been mistreated). It may appear that parents aren't listening, but when problems become serious, standard parenting techniques of negotiation and responsive listening may be inadequate. Teachers, school counselors, therapists, clergy, social service workers, and others often concentrate exclusively on trying to convey understanding of adolescents' feelings, a compassionate approach that, unfortunately, may make some problems worse.

The triangles formed by uncontrolled young people and various adult "authority" figures, anxious to appear understanding, create cross-genera-tional coalitions that only increase the rebellious power these kids wield. Even therapists—presumed experts on the human scene—still have a tendency to identify children as victims of repressive parental authority and to keep parents at arm's length (except, of course, when it comes to presenting the bill).

Individual therapy with aggressive young people is associated with notoriously poor outcome. Systemic family therapists may become para-lyzed when dealing with hard-core hard-to-manage teens because of a lack of motivation on the part of beleaguered parents too worn down to keep fighting. What, then, is an effective approach to working with difficult adolescents?

THE HUMANIST APPROACH

The need for both kindness and authority requires that the problem of youthful aggression be approached from both a strategic and a humanistic perspective. Humanism is an old and venerable approach to life. The humanist movement came into being in the United States in the early 1900s. One of its founders was Corliss Lamont, who became a director of the American Civil Liberties Union and an honorary President of the American Humanist Association. His book *Philosophy of Humanism* (1990) is still a primary source for understanding the concepts of secular humanism. The humanistic movement continues to flourish and has permeated the field of psychotherapy (which always seems to be strug-gling to find philosophical underpinnings). In the 1960s humanistic psychology emerged as a popular protest against such approaches as psychoanalysis and behaviorism. The following quote from a position paper issued by the Association for Humanistic Psychology (1987) ex-plains this emergence from the point of view of humanistic psychologists:

> During the first half of the twentieth century, American psychology was dominated by two schools of thought: behaviorism and psychoanalysis. Neither fully acknowledged the possibility of studying values, intentions and meaning as elements in conscious existence. Although various Euro-pean perspectives such as phenomenology had some limited influence, on the whole mainstream American psychology had been captured by the mechanistic beliefs of behaviorism and by the biological reductionism and determinism of classical psychoanalysis.
>
> By the late 1950s a "Third Force" was beginning to form. In 1957 and 1958, at the invitation of Abraham Maslow and Clark Moustakas, two

meetings were held in Detroit among psychologists who were interested in founding a professional association dedicated to a more meaningful, more humanistic vision. They discussed several themes—such as self, self-actualization, health, creativity, intrinsic nature, being, becoming, individuality, and meaning—which they believed likely to become central concerns of such an approach to psychology.

At a time in history when our society was moving toward a focus on love and emotional expression, humanistic psychotherapy pushed for an understanding of the person as a self-directed being who has free will and can solve problems. Now that three more decades have passed, humanistic psychology has fallen out of fashion but continues to have a core of adherents and something to say to us all. The fall from mainstream popularity of humanistic psychology can be attributed, at least in part, to its earlier emphasis on ideology over concrete clinical technique. Today, in our impatience with approaches that seem to be all heart and no head, we may be in danger of practicing just the reverse—emphasizing technique without compassion. We mustn't lose sight of the essence of humanistic psychology.

In the last 20 years humanistic institutes, offering M.A. and Ph.D. Degrees in humanistic psychology, have sprung up across the country. There are now thousands of therapists who formally identify themselves as humanistic. This proliferation of humanistic psychology has led many people to wonder what makes this philosophy so attractive.

Humanism and Control over One's Destiny

The strength of humanism lies in its belief in the individual and in the individual's ability to control his or her own destiny. Central to humanism is the belief that people aren't the hapless victims of fate, emotional disease, or genetics but can use their minds and their hearts in harmony to rise above their circumstances. However, humanism's basically nondirective style doesn't offer much concrete guidance to the therapist on harnessing this mind–heart coalition. Humanistic psychology, like feminism, is not a set of techniques; it is a sensibility that informs clinical work. Whether they choose to practice psychoanalysis or behavior therapy, all humanistic therapists are guided by a belief in the fundamental goodness of people, in our ultimate responsibility to take charge of our own lives, and in our duty to live up to our obligations to others.

The strategic approach put forth in these chapters is both directive and humanistic. This highly technical approach is informed by a humanistic concern for individuals—with all their rights and responsibilities.

Humanism versus Determinism

In every therapist's career a decision must be made between humanistic and deterministic philosophies. A humanist believes in the resilience of the human spirit and the ability of the human mind to solve problems; a determinist understands symptoms as being outside the control of the client and may refer to the occurrence of similar symptoms in a parent and grandparent as evidence of predetermination. Humanists are likely to see emotional symptoms as attempts to solve problems in life whereas determinists are more likely to see symptoms as biochemical events, disease, or deeply ingrained psychopathology.

Emotional symptoms must be seen as either within or outside the control of the individual. This dichotomy between humanistic and deterministic perspectives usually manifests itself as a schism between nondirective and directive approaches to therapy. Although humanists are typically seen as nondirective (whereas directive therapists are expected to be coldhearted "button pushers"), the strategic approach presented in these pages is both humanistic and directive.

THE QUESTION OF TECHNIQUE

Humanism in therapy, though philosophically important, needs help when it comes to technique. Technique is critical when serious symptoms like violence and aggression must be treated. The first priority in dealing with an emergency is immediate and constructive action. There's nothing inherently contradictory between decisiveness and humanism. From a strategic humanistic position, the questions are: How does a therapist intervene effectively in a crisis in a way that helps each person's potential come to light? Must all methods appear sweetly reasonable and philosophically correct, or should we be more concerned with creating conditions that bring out the best in each person's self-directive nature? May therapists let their power to help people show while also being compassionate? How does a therapist intervene forcefully *and* in a way that's compassionate and humane?

Any way of helping people that moves them in the direction of greater self-determination, self-respect, and skill in solving their own problems can be defined as humane. Methods that seek to understand human nature and then use that knowledge to bring out the good, the compassionate, and the forgiving in people can also be defined as humane. I regard any process that uses deliberate action and intervention to increase the existence of generous and compassionate interaction between people as humane.

As a strategic family therapist and teacher of family therapists, I've often observed that most therapy is accomplished in the first two sessions. When treating aggressive adolescents, the therapist must rapidly instill hope in those initial sessions by communicating a clear view of change. In my time spent with Jay Haley and Cloé Madanes, I've been most impressed by the way they organized these first few moments of therapy. Seasoned therapists seem to have an innate sense of the need in clients for hope, for a sense of there being light at the end of the tunnel. I began to focus on trying to understand how that hope is generated. It isn't always obvious. How do people coming to therapists with so much pain take hope or inspiration without feeling that their concerns are being minimized? The answer lies in helping people find a sense of direction—even when they feel lost.

In the Disney movie of A. A. Milne's "Winnie the Pooh and Tigger Too," Pooh, Rabbit, and Tigger are lost in the woods in a deep fog. Rabbit, a sparkling example of our average human, keeps heading for home and repeatedly finds himself, with his friends in tow, back at the same sand pit. Despite his repeated failure, Rabbit says, "It's lucky I know these woods so well or we might get lost." Pooh, in his characteristic "brainless" and very human way suggests, "Rabbit, how about if when we get out of sight of this old pit we just try to find it again? When we look for home we keep finding this pit. So I thought that if we looked for this pit we might find home." Pooh's words of wisdom fall on deaf ears as Rabbit offers to demonstrate that if he tries to find the pit again, he will surely find it. Rabbit wanders off to dramatize his point and never returns. What would have given Rabbit enough hope to believe that an illogical idea like Pooh's just might begin to break down an unfortunate repetitive cycle of pain and fear? How could Pooh have presented his idea, had he been a therapist, so that Rabbit would have seen a light? Or could Pooh have simply directed the group's actions in such a way that they found home whether Rabbit understood the strange logic of it or not?

Helping Families Find Hope

Families asking for help with out-of-control adolescents and young adults are often lost in fog-shrouded woods with frightening, shadowy specters all around them. Unfortunately, many of these specters—violence, arrest, drug abuse, dissolution of the family—are quite real. The therapist's ability to help transform these dark possibilities into happy, successful outcomes is his or her greatest power and gift.

The approach in this book emphasizes what's needed in therapy to lead people in the direction of hope and healing, a direction that, although certainly not the end of the job, turns out to be both essential and profound. My task is to clarify how to help families break free of despair. How do therapists understand people's dilemmas in ways that generate creative growth and self-determination? How does a therapist speak in ways that inspire and initiate change? With the family's center of gravity shifted slightly off center, how do we choose directives and tasks that act as fulcrums in levering people toward new, creative directions?

Do people want to change? Certainly they do. Even the angriest and most self-destructive adolescent wants to be a better and more responsible person. The tenacity of an anorexic's sickness or of a bad actor's bad attitude may make them seem unwilling to change or oblivious to efforts to get through to them. But experience tells me they aren't. They're afraid.

One reason family therapists encounter so much resistance is that they're too eager to change people and too slow to understand them. Family therapists learn to accurately see as circular a wife's nagging and a husband's withdrawal, but they've been slow to see these behaviors as human, slow to see through the nagging to the pain behind it, and slow to understand the anxiety that motivates the withdrawal.

The power to work effectively with tough cases in family therapy, which I hope you will discover in these pages, comes from a combination of caring and confrontation, with the former helping to make the latter possible. Families, like individuals, resist efforts to change them by people they feel don't understand and accept them. Each chapter in this book explains and demonstrates rapidly and in broad strokes an approach that helps organize cases of severely acting out and aggressive young people.

I was educated in graduate school as a behaviorist. With an interest in transactional analysis and Gestalt psychology, I was supervised by a psychoanalyst and attempted to do psychoanalytic therapy with inner-city heroin addicts. Despite these confusing beginnings, I've always gravitated toward techniques and understandings that bring about rapid change.

When I began my practice in community mental health in 1978, I was immediately uncomfortable and quite confused about the view of clients and their problems I'd been taught, namely, that people are disturbed and passive participants in a process of mental illness. At first I didn't like my clients and therapy was a chore. I viewed my clients as opponents too handicapped to realize that they were making terrible mistakes. Many were "passive–aggressive," and my job was to convince them that they were doing bad things. I'd try to listen sincerely with deep empathy for their plight but would become angry when my compassion didn't inspire them to turn over a new leaf.

Therapeutic Approaches

As I looked for practical and benevolent approaches to treatment, I was introduced to the work of Salvador Minuchin and Jay Haley; later I discovered the work of Cloé Madanes. Minuchin's approach was dynamic and brief, but my sense was that he believed people were ruled by the structure of their families (Minuchin, 1974). He didn't seem sure that people wanted to change. His focus on the controlling power of subsystems and boundaries seemed to emphasize why people stayed the same more than it showed ways they could change. While Minuchin taught me that therapists could be powerful and take an active role in helping people change, I still felt some of the old sense that my clients were opponents and that I had to push, shock, or cajole them into changing.

Haley and Madanes introduced me to a related approach with a different twist. They worked from the assumption that people want to change and that they develop symptoms in an attempt to help those they love. This was what I'd been waiting to hear. I still thought about hierarchy and family structure, but now I felt freer to like my clients.

Practicing in community mental health clinics, I found myself challenged to succeed but expected to fail. The staff would refer me those cases other therapists felt were hopeless, with family therapy being viewed as the treatment of last resort. As a result, my caseload became predominantly violent couples and acting-out teenagers. I realized later that those tough cases were a gift. Helping aggressive adolescents and violent couples enabled me to feel certain I'd influenced someone's life for the better.

Working with Madanes and Haley, I focused on refining a therapeutic approach with difficult teenagers and their families. During years of experience with a great many cases, I noticed a general direction for therapy that, when followed, usually made things come out well. Paradoxically, this approach often required me to be at odds with the kinds of teenagers I'd befriended during my first years of individual therapy practice. I came to understand that being forceful was necessary to help young people change—and to help their families change with them. Despite how uncomfortable it felt being unpopular with some of my teenage clients, I decided to do what worked—and to learn to become comfortable with it.

Since all human interactions are a series of maneuvers (Haley, 1976), therapy can be seen as a series of organizational strategies meant to transform the painful realities clients bring to therapy. Any statement by a therapist is an intervention. Therefore, it follows that if therapists understand how their interventions have changed an individual client's experience or a family's interactions, they'll be able to replicate those approaches in the future. Intentionally intervening to help people resolve painful symptoms involves the use of both power and compassion.

When helping parents or caretakers regain control of their families, therapists must feel free to exercise power. They can then empower parents to transform painful realities into a context in which they can again feel love and compassion for their children. Just as we ask parents to discover their courage, so too must therapists be courageous enough to take powerful action despite their own anxieties. Like the people they work with, therapists often feel controlled and helpless. This is not because they're victims of family folly and deceit but because they don't understand the forces that pit husbands and wives and parents and children against each other. As a result, therapists, just like average men and women, are all too often ready to blame and vilify. Blaming is a refuge for feeling helpless.

When families come to me for help, I assume they have problems not because there is something inherently wrong with them but because they've simply gotten stuck either with a structure whose time has passed or with a story that doesn't work. This perspective, of course, highlights the difference between the therapist, who merely *observes* family interactions, and family members, who are *living* those interactions. What keeps people stuck is the great difficulty they have in seeing their own participation in the problems that plague them. With their eyes fixed firmly on what those recalcitrant others are doing, it's hard for most people to see the patterns that bind them together. Part of my job is to give them a wake-up call—but without throwing cold water on them.

The familiar image of the therapist—kindly, benevolent, and relatively silent—is based on the psychoanalytic model of discovering meaning in the client's words in a thoughtful, leisurely process. I want to prepare you for a very different kind of therapy.

FINDING NEW SOLUTIONS

In the pages that follow, you will see ordinary men and women wrestling with difficulties that have gotten the best of them. You'll hear their words and sense their heartache; often you'll know how they feel. What you may not always see, however, is the incredible pressure people feel to keep using old solutions.

For all their uncertainty, kindness, and vulnerability, families are rigidly organized and their members are frightened of the unknown—especially in those areas where they are bogged down in problems. I care about people, but as a therapist I'm not content just to be understanding. I want to help people break out of their cycles of self-defeating behavior.

At times, when family members can't see their part in maintaining problems or aren't willing to take the risk to try solutions they don't understand, there appears to be a struggle between them and me. The therapy process I describe in this book sometimes takes on the appearance of sparring. When I say to a father that he's not doing enough or tell a mother that she's unwittingly excluding her husband, it may seem as if there's a struggle between the client and me or as if I'm attacking the client. But I don't think of it that way. From my perspective, the struggle is between me and the clients' hopelessness and fear—fear of change.

At the heart of this book is a paradigm that views the parents of aggressive adolescents as abuse victims rather than as victimizers. The adolescents whose lives are explored in these chapters are often victims as well, despite the fact that they're stuck in the role of abuser in many cases. I begin by discussing the causes of parent abuse and then describe identifiable patterns in the interactions of family members trapped in the nightmare that emerges when parents feel victimized by their children.

ONE

Parent Abuse

UNDERSTANDING EMOTIONAL ABUSE

Emotional abuse is an abstraction that's hard to define. The concept of emotional abuse developed from the idea that human beings can use their knowledge of the weaknesses of others to control, dominate, or exploit them. When one person knows that another is in a weakened emotional state and utilizes that weakness to take advantage of that person, such behavior qualifies as abuse.

As an example of emotional abuse, consider the following scenario: A single mother who is overweight views herself as fat, unattractive, and weak-willed. One day her 13-year-old son asks if he can go to a rock concert that would keep him out until 2:00 A.M. His mother says no. The boy accuses his mother of wanting him home early only because she's using him for company. Seeing her blanch, he goes on to say that she just wants to run his life because she can't control her own. The elements that make the boy's response abusive, rather than just rude, are revealed in an examination of the emotional content of this interaction. The son's allusions to his mother's weight and self-doubt put her in a position of needing to defend not only her concerns about his staying out late but also her character, a position that leads to confusion on her part. While his mother is confused about her right to complain about her son's hours, the boy attacks her in an area where she's most vulnerable. Her doubts about both her attractiveness and her competence as a mother are used to incapacitate her emotionally. In two sentences the boy has invoked her self-doubt, shame, and fear of losing his love in his effort to block her attempts to exercise reasonable control. When the son brings up an area of concern that isn't related to the hours he keeps, he is manipulating his mother's emotions to such an extent that she can no longer tell whether her personal characteristics are relevant to the argument or not. The mother then withdraws, feeling humiliated, weak, ashamed, and confused about how such feelings could come out of a simple statement that staying out until 2:00 A.M. isn't acceptable.

Clinical Vignette

A more detailed vignette from my clinical practice provides further illustration of the most common forms of abuse perpetrated by teens and young adults against their parents. In this case tactics similar to those described above are used by adolescents when a conversation isn't going their way.

An urban North Carolina family, the Baldwins, were seen at a community mental health center after being referred by the local hospital, to which the oldest of the two daughters was admitted after a trip to the emergency room. Lisa and Jean were 14 and 16 years old, respectively. Both had made serious suicide attempts by drug overdose in the 6 months before their mother brought them for therapy. Mr. and Mrs. Baldwin were divorced; they were openly angry and were still struggling in court over money.

My conversation with the family began with my explaining why I hadn't had any luck getting the girls' father to come in for a session, either separately or with his ex-wife and daughters. Mr. Baldwin had agreed to attend sessions but hadn't shown up at the scheduled times. In view of the danger to his daughters, I decided that Mr. Baldwin's lack of involvement had to be confronted. The need to contact him was punctuated by his daughters' insistence on speaking for him in sessions and defending him. Despite Mrs. Baldwin's verbal assaults on him (and his girlfriend) and her legal actions against him, it was beginning to look as if Mr. Baldwin was the more troubled parent. When I discussed his indifference toward his children, Mrs. Baldwin agreed with me. Their daughters then attempted what they did at home: They tried to emotionally neutralize their mother so that she wouldn't give up on making him look good through her questionable acts.

Lisa, a tall dark-haired beauty, sat pensively between her mother and her older sister. Jean leaned toward Lisa and directed an angry, haughty look toward their mother. Mrs. Baldwin was young and attractive, with auburn hair, but she had a sheepish look about her. I began feeling slightly daunted by the teenagers, who were sending a lot of nonverbal messages back and forth; I had the impression that they were in charge of their rather apologetic mother because their manner so dominated the therapy room.

Thinking that perhaps an assault on her ex-husband, with whom she was so angry, would help Mrs. Baldwin display some evidence that she was in control, I said to her, "The girls keep avoiding the subject when we discuss anything about their father. Frankly, I think they're protecting him. I'm curious about why they explode whenever I get close to getting him involved."

Lisa, staring plaintively at her mother, responded, "We already told him. He doesn't . . . he's not in our immediate family; I mean, he is our immediate family—"

"He's your father!" Mrs. Baldwin interrupted.

This was confusing. The girls seemed to be discounting the importance of their father while his angry ex-wife appeared to be defending him. I was hoping that Mrs. Baldwin would take the position that her ex-husband wasn't doing his job and that it was her job (and mine) to get him to participate. In order to draw a line defining Mrs. Baldwin as the mother, it seemed necessary that I scold Jean and Lisa for being disrespectful toward her. "Wait a minute," I stated emphatically. "I'm not asking for your explanation of why your father—"

I was interrupted by Lisa, who threw up her hand and laughingly proclaimed, "I believe you."

Jean finally chimed in. "Yeah, we believe you," she said in a sarcastic tone of voice.

"It's important that you hear this," I tried again, sounding a bit more irritated.

"No, it's not!" Jean said, angrily continuing to block my attempts to discuss her father.

Once again I tried to act as if Mrs. Baldwin was the head of the family: I addressed her in a manner that suggested that I believed she had knowledge the girls lacked. "I'd like you to tell me a little more . . . you know him in a way that they don't."

"Yeah," she answered halfheartedly.

Lisa, usually the quiet one, laughed in her mother's face after hearing her lack of conviction. Jean looked at Lisa, then glanced at her mother, then looked back at Lisa and smiled at her with a condescending roll of her eyes toward Mrs. Baldwin. Despite this setback, I tried to use Mrs. Baldwin's status to define her as knowledgeable. "You were his wife, after all."

"Yeah," she again answered halfheartedly. I groaned inwardly, knowing that Mrs. Baldwin had just invited her daughters to begin another verbal barrage.

Lisa yelled out, "You don't know him anymore." Jean responded nonverbally by smiling and playfully slapping at her sister, encouraging her to go on. Lisa rose to the challenge and exclaimed in a sarcastic snarl, "After all, he's not your type."

I attempted to take direct control. "Listen," I said, "I'm sure you girls will have comments to make when we're—"

Mrs. Baldwin rose to the occasion by interrupting me and snapping, "Could you at least be courteous?" to Lisa and Jean.

Undaunted, Lisa simply said, "No."

I continued where I left off: "But right now, I'm going to ask you to listen very carefully and be sure to note anything you're going to want to straighten out afterwards, okay?"

Surprisingly, Lisa said, "Okay."

Jean joined her with, "Yeah."

I was thinking that sometimes a therapist has to be as stubborn and persistent as a teenager, so I picked up where I left off earlier and asked Mrs. Baldwin, "What happens with their father when it gets close to him coming in for an appointment and he fails that? I intentionally set it up so that he could come at a separate time when nobody else was here and he still didn't come in." Jean leaned back in her chair, dramatically throwing her head back and rolling her eyes, as if to say, "What a load of garbage"; but she didn't speak.

Mrs. Baldwin followed my lead of not responding to the girls and said, "I don't think Harold really believes in therapy, at all, basically. For some reason, it's getting too close to him. He has his own therapist that he has been going to off and on, but he goes maybe once every 2 weeks or once every 3 weeks."

This was material that may have been new to the daughters. If so, I reasoned, they might listen attentively to a discussion on the subject of their father's therapy. I asked, "What is he seeing a therapist for?"

Mrs. Baldwin responded, "I don't even know anymore. It started with a lot to do with himself. I think getting through the divorce and all kind of things; they were trying to help him that way. But he's got a wall, and he doesn't like anybody real, real close to him."

Again, a critical comment about their father was sufficient to trigger the girls' attempts to stop their mother from speaking decisively about their father. Jean leaned toward Mrs. Baldwin and screamed, "Oh, bull-shit."

Almost simultaneously Lisa yelled, "Oh really?"

Mrs. Baldwin looked at me and, her previous feeble tone of voice returning, said, "Yeah."

Jean escalated the hostility further by yelling, "Go ask Lydia."

Mocking her mother, Lisa shouted, "Yeah, go ask Lydia."

While Mrs. Baldwin described her ex-husband, the girls nonverbally provided the atmosphere of a circus. The more the discussion threatened to discredit their father, the more emotionally assaultive they became toward their mother. This disrespectful mood remained nonverbal until they began attacking their mother with details of their father's relationship with a new woman; they did this knowing that their mother had never really recovered from the divorce. Despite Lisa and Jean's determination to disable their mother's resolve, I continued to discuss Mr. Baldwin. I intended in this way to initiate a crisis in which either Mrs. Baldwin would rise to the occasion and handle her daughters or the girls would at least realize that the adults were aware of the covert assistance they were giving their father and would perhaps consider other methods for helping him.

The session continued with the girls challenging their mother about her actions which provided covert support for her ex-husband by acting irrationally and thereby making him look good. Such acts included repeatedly phoning her ex-husband and then hanging up, as well as searching his office when the girls were there cleaning for him. The girls continued to use the single technique of defending their father and blaming their mother for all the family's ills in the family situation. I was thrilled when Mrs. Baldwin found some inner reserve of strength and with dignity told her daughters, "Well, maybe he does let the wall down for her, I don't know. But that's still my opinion." Lisa seemed surprised by this comment and merely mumbled under her breath. Seeing that she might be gaining some leverage, Mrs. Baldwin continued, "But as far as the children are concerned, I don't understand him because they are his kids and I don't understand why he wouldn't want to help them."

At this point Jean, who had assumed a closed posture in which she seemed to be curling into herself, head toward knees, raised her head and in a voice devoid of conviction said, "We don't have any problems with him."

Now that the balance of power appeared to be shifting toward Mrs. Baldwin, I said, "Mrs. Baldwin, to change the subject for just a minute . . . how's Jean doing with her problem of overeating and throwing up?" I was hoping that by diverting the discussion to Jean and Lisa as patients, they wouldn't change the subject and resume their attack on their mother. Both girls became more serious and allowed this discussion to continue without interrupting.

After a discussion of eating and throwing up, the two girls, who were now sitting facing each other, began giggling as I spoke to Mrs. Baldwin. "I'm going to push harder to get Harold to come in," I said, "and for the two of you to talk about your daughters' problems and find some solutions. How do you think their father is doing since the divorce?"

Lisa answered, "Great."

Jean added, "Pretty good."

Mrs. Baldwin repeated, "Pretty good." Then she continued, saying, "I think he's pretty happy."

At this point Lisa changed the subject, directing the discussion away from her father by offering to make herself the patient: "He's happy, but I'm not."

Children's feelings and symptoms are a powerful diversion. They offer interesting information that a therapist may choose to pursue. Despite the temptation to ask why Lisa wasn't happy, I again stuck to my intention of being as stubborn as a teenager and continued my focus on Mr. Baldwin: "One of the reasons he may be so happy is because the things that you've done out of your anger really make him look like a saint."

Mrs. Baldwin again surprised me with her strength by answering, "That's probably true."

I continued, "He really comes off looking good—too good. It doesn't add up. Nobody's that good. Everybody's convinced that he's just wonderful. Even you're convinced."

Mrs. Baldwin weakly responded, "No . . . not anymore."

Since directly discussing Mr. Baldwin had resulted in the daughters' attacking their mother, I was wondering if shifting the responsibility for family problems to their mother might bring out a more supportive side of the girls. Mrs. Baldwin wasn't convincing in expressing her belief that her ex-husband bore some responsibility for the family's difficulties, so I had to push harder to get her to make a statement with some conviction. "You divorced the man and you're convinced."

With a little more conviction this time, she said, "No, I'm not going to see him as wonderful anymore." Lisa broke out laughing, but Mrs. Baldwin, who was warming to the experience of being more powerful, asserted, "I think he's shirking his responsibility with the kids."

As Mrs. Baldwin began acting more convinced of her ex-husband's weaknesses, she also spoke about her acceptance of the divorce. Her growing acceptance of the divorce threatened the balance her daughters maintained by protecting their father. That is, the girls' involvement in the postdivorce struggle kept their parents joined together, albeit angrily; however, it also prevented them from dealing with each other directly.

One after the other, Lisa and Jean shouted, "He is not!" Their mother's assertion that their father was shirking his duty was underscored by the fact that both suicide attempts had been made at his house. In addition, he'd been unsympathetic toward the girls' emotional concerns and had spent little time at the hospital when they were admitted for the suicide attempts. The girls' litany of abuse continued, with Jean looking at me and yelling, "He doesn't know."

Lisa echoed, "You don't know anything, Mom! He's changed. She doesn't know him anymore." As Lisa tried to redirect her mother, she was anxiously leaning forward and running her fingers through her hair.

I pushed further, linking the family struggle to the need for Mr. Baldwin to be protected. "I think the struggle that happens in this family with you three helps him maintain his wonderfulness," I told them.

Mrs. Baldwin leaned forward and asked, "What do I need to do?"

As her mother's resolve became stronger, Lisa began a more aggressive escalation of emotionally abusive tactics. "So you think my father is totally bad or something? My father—you don't understand! (*to mother*) You don't understand! (*to me*) My mother isn't around my father anymore. My dad has changed. My dad is in love with someone else, and Mom can't accept it! I don't care what she says. She'll say she doesn't love my father anymore. I told you that, and she'll get all upset. I'm sick and tired of it!" Lisa angrily pointed her finger at her mother during her lengthy exclamation.

Now the other half of the team, Jean, yelled, "Well, she went out the door last night calling his girlfriend a shit and a cunt, that—"

Like a tag-team wrestler who just got called back into the ring, Lisa now took up the attack by screaming, "He'll always love you as a person, but *can't you accept that he's not in love with you anymore?*"

Mrs. Baldwin had again succumbed to the attack and was doubled up, her head in her hands. She feebly responded, "Yes, I can."

Lisa countered, "No, you can't!"

Like a child losing an argument with a sibling, repeating her words but betraying by her tone of voice her lack of confidence in her position, Mrs. Baldwin again replied, "Yes, I can."

Seeing an opportunity to make her mother the problem instead of her father, Lisa kept driving her point home. She yelled, "Where do you get off lying and saying you don't grill us all the time? You do!"

Mrs. Baldwin again responded weakly, this time with, "I don't grill you all the time. I asked you about Thanksgiving." Mrs. Baldwin was losing ground rapidly because she was responding to the content of her daughters' accusations. She was missing the point by not realizing that she wasn't answerable to them about her handling of adult relationships. As Mrs. Baldwin failed to correct Lisa and Jean for speaking to her that way, her daughters' hostility escalated. She had trouble stopping them because she knew that much of what they were saying was true.

Lisa continued, "Last night, you even said that she was a shit and a cunt. He's our dad, and Lydia's our friend."

The girls' verbal abuse was keeping their mother in a defensive position at the same time that it sustained her anger toward them. In a sense, the abuse made her stronger by fueling her emotional intensity, which in turn demonstrated that in her mind the marriage wasn't yet over. Mrs. Baldwin really was mishandling her ex-husband, but an acceptance of the fact that she needed to change her behavior toward him required her to admit that her marriage was truly over.

After choreographing a struggle in the therapy room that dramatized how painful the relationships in the family had become, I was now ready to demonstrate to Mrs. Baldwin that even terrible verbal abuse by children could still be the result of their feelings of compassion and protectiveness. I finally remarked to her, "It's sort of like arguing with your husband, isn't it?"

Mrs. Baldwin responded quietly, "Yeah," as tears welled up in her eyes.

I ordinarily wouldn't encourage a single parent to collapse in tears in front of her children when she needs to be strong. However, Mrs. Baldwin's apparent strength was unconvincing, and I was hoping that this display of her true pain might elicit a kindly side of the girls. As their mother broke down instead of reacting angrily, Lisa and Jean began to change. Neither daughter had spoken while her mother was so upset. As I continued to point out Mrs. Baldwin's helpfulness to her ex-husband, Lisa and Jean left their seats and walked across the room toward their mother. Each gave her mother a kiss and told her that she loved her. The girls then left the office—as if to say, "Okay, we'll let you help her now."

It is often the case that confronting the adolescent's abusive behavior rather than allowing it to continue, makes it possible for the benevolent feelings in the adolescent to surface. In the case of the Baldwins, that confrontation destroyed the illusion that Lisa and Jean were abusive and cruel.

EMOTIONAL BLACKMAIL

Parent abuse includes forms of emotional blackmail such as the following:

- Threats of impending physical assault
- Threats of suicide
- Threats of such self-destructive acts as quitting school, running away, using drugs, and indiscriminate sex
- *The hammer of the '90s:* Threats of reporting parents to child protective services for any physical restraint or aggression utilized in response to abusive behavior
- Provocation by vulgarity and personal attack to bring about inappropriate adult responses

As we explore the different forms of emotional abuse used by adolescents and young adults, it will become clear that there is some overlap between categories. Some illustrations of emotional abuse have characteristics of more than one kind of threat. For example, a teenager who provokes a parent by vulgarity and personal attack until the parent says something cruel may then respond by threatening suicide.

VERBAL EMOTIONAL ABUSE:
THE NEGOTIATIONS BEGIN WITH "NO"

Among the most common forms of emotional abuse against parents is the language-based approach. Parents begin their attempts to get adolescents to listen to adult reason with a distinct disadvantage. Cultural prescriptions have defined proper parenting for the parents of today, and children use some of these generalizations about what constitutes appropriate parenting to effectively criticize their parents. Criticism by teenagers of their parents often involves such catchphrases as the following:

♦ "Children must make their own mistakes."
♦ "If parents take charge, young people will never learn responsibility themselves."
♦ "Children must learn responsibility by being left alone and not interfered with."
♦ "It's their life."
♦ "Children must be trusted [whether they've earned that trust or not]; otherwise, the growth of the inner self will be stunted and creativity and self-expression thwarted."
♦ "Parents should always explain themselves to their children."
♦ "Young people have to make their own decisions" (therefore, parents shouldn't force their judgment on young people).
♦ "Children shouldn't be told what to do" (because they'll come to resent their parents, and their rebelliousness will be the parents' fault).
♦ "A child's ego will be harmed if his or her right to total privacy is violated."
♦ "It's intrusive to punish without giving advance warning as to the consequence."

These platitudes, though useful in some cases, became accepted truths in the permissive climate of the 1960s and '70s. In those years our society was struggling to come out of an era that had been ruled by a view of children as the property of adults. Children had few rights, and parents could do almost anything they wished to their children without repercussions. Forms of child rearing were then proposed that emphasized recognition of the child's feelings. This "humanizing" of children was an important step toward an acceptance of the concept of children's rights.

The new ethics in child rearing that evolved in the 1960s and '70s primarily stressed children's needs, but the focus shifted away from the need for structure and leadership and emphasized kindness as a panacea. The belief in the importance of heeding children's opinions on decisions that affected them came to be sacrosanct. Children's behaviors were seen as the manifestation of feelings, and the importance of expressing those feelings became the central theme of positive parenting. The elixir that would cure all childhood ills was parental respect for the child's need for "attention." Even in the '90s parents often come in for therapy saying that they think their child is "just trying to get attention." Yet these parents are confused because they also understand that their child has become the family's primary focus of attention. The child's behavioral problems are attributed to the absence of such primary ingredients as love, a mother at home, an altruistic brother or sister, or a male role model. Something positive and loving is seen as missing. This reductionistic view of a child's behavioral problems derives from the belief that parental cruelty, autocracy, and lack of concern about children's feelings are the main reasons children become emotionally disturbed.

Stated simply, the rule that has come to dominate today's theories of child rearing is that parents must be lenient. Parents of difficult children are scolded for being too strict or closed-minded. The apparent strictness of these chastised parents is inferred from their rigid, angry, inflexible statements. When the actual behavior of these "strict" parents is observed, however, they are often found to be quite incapable of getting their children to live by the rules they expound. In other words, they talk tough but act lenient.

Rather than leniency being the expression of parental love, in practice it may express the opposite. When they take firm and loving control of their children, parents are more likely to be in a position to love their children openly and easily. When this firm and loving control is done well, there are fewer destructive battles for control that no one ever really wins. With less anger and fewer arguments, both parents and teens feel more kindly toward each other and there's more compassion to go around. Children feel more secure when they get a sense of strength coming from the people who are there to care for them and keep them safe.

There has been an indiscriminate application by some helping professionals of philosophies that are inappropriate to certain populations. So too there is an uncritical application to the raising of troubled children of parenting ideas that were developed for use with normal children. Regardless of how disturbed a young person might be, a single set of child-rearing guidelines is expected to hold true. For instance, experts say to trust your children. Yet trust might not be wise when your child is known to torture animals and steal from stores. When a child throws clichés from "experts" in a parent's face, that child may gain power and increase his or her ability to be verbally and emotionally abusive.

Tactics that attack parents by using the gospel according to the "experts" are particularly effective in an era that has spawned the self-help movement. That movement has generated such parent categories as "toxic parents" and "adult children of dysfunctional parents." These and other self-help concepts reinforce the idea that all problems in the present can be explained by damage done in the past, and parents are routinely blamed for all difficulties their children encounter. Self-help books and programs should be approached with caution. Their concepts are *suggestions* that may offer direction to those venturing into the world of personal growth and change. These programs often achieve a bad reputation when certain acolytes begin a mission to show others that their ideas must be true for all people.

More and more problems of childhood and young adulthood are being explained by blaming parents. Parents are vulnerable to feelings of guilt at all times. These feelings are particularly strong if children aren't turning out the way their parents had hoped. Guilt over being a poor parent is exacerbated by a society that's forcing more and more parents out of the home. In an economy designed for two-income households, not only are parents around less but their functions are being usurped by social agencies such as schools, churches, day-care centers, and the courts. The assumption now seems to be that children won't receive an adequate education or set of values at home. Courses on values clarification and human sexuality are taught in most schools. Though useful, these programs are part of a trend that undermines parents. Children are bonding to teachers in school or to coaches and instructors in after-school programs and asking their parents why they can't be more like these new role models. Children are forming groups in schools for every possible childhood problem—divorced parents, gay and lesbian interests, alcoholism in the family, and so on—and parents are rarely invited to attend these meetings. In general, society is turning away from the parents as the principal guides in a child's development. The situation is even worse for single parents who often feel so unsupported and blamed that they may spoil a child, to make up for the inequities resulting from the loss or lack of a second parent, rather than be firm.

Despite the usefulness of many programs, groups, and services for youth, their proliferation indicates a frightening direction for our culture. Is it the chicken or the egg? Because parents feel more and more disenfranchised, they leave parenting to public agencies and professionals. The more they hand over their authority to others, the more disenfranchised they feel. This surrender of parental authority is like a runaway train threatening the very lives it was designed to help.

There's a lot of talk these days about "dysfunctional families" as a source of human unhappiness. Unfortunately, much of this talk amounts to little more than parent bashing. Children's suffering is viewed as the result of what their parents do—or fail to do. A mother's career, a father's brutish ways, a parent's drinking—these are the causes of all the trouble young people get into. Perhaps this is better than demonizing troubled teens themselves, but it's a long way from understanding what really goes on in families. One reason for blaming family sorrows on the personal failings of parents is that it's very hard for the average person to see past individual personalities to the structural patterns that make up a family and to view the family as a system of interconnected lives governed by strict but unspoken rules.

Understanding the trend toward parent blaming makes it easier to recognize the abusive negotiation techniques often employed by adolescents. In healthy families, parents explain their decisions to their children to a reasonable extent. These explanations lead to discussions that clarify what the parents mean and may clarify what the young person agrees or disagrees with. Then, using the information from these discussions, parents will either change their position or stick with their original decision. That ends the negotiation. Abusive young people demand that parents explain their decisions only for the purpose of gathering enough information to use as ammunition in their struggle to convince their parents that they are acting like adults who are either crazy, unreasonable, out of touch with the times, or just plain mean. The choice of accusation depends on what the young person knows will best arouse the guilt of the parent. The following sequence illustrates the basic steps in the development of an abusive conversation:

1. The young person makes a request.
2. The parent asks for information clarifying details of the request.
3. The young person responds courteously and provides the information.
4. The parent acknowledges the child's point of view but says that the child may not have permission to do what was asked. (Ordinarily this is the point where a discussion would still be possible. This discussion could lead to a compromise, or at least to an agreement on how such a request could be handled the next time it's made. For instance, a parent might agree that a request was reasonable but say that not enough notice was given.)
5. The young person now attempts to change the parent's resolve by reasoning. He or she asks for more details on the parent's rationale for the decision. However, the purpose of this request isn't to understand what the parent thinks; it is an attempt to gather information that can be used to argue with the parent's reasoning. The child continues challenging parental logic until he or she is convinced that the decision isn't going to change.

6. The young person then begins a series of vociferous abusive remarks designed to exasperate the parent until he or she gives in. This abusive technique requires that the young person pursue the outcome relentlessly and not give up until the battle is won. The relentlessness may involve following a parent around as he or she tries to get away from the screaming attack. Parents have been known to lock themselves in the bathroom out of sheer frustration.

When the screaming begins and the defending follows, any hope of communicating ends. Seeing each other's point of view is no longer the issue. The argument becomes a battle of wills resulting in a winner and a loser. The winner is established as right and the loser as wrong. Each sentence uttered is formulated to disqualify the opinion of the opponent. Despite pleas from parents and teens for respect and fairness, there's none to be found in such an interaction. The talk rapidly degenerates into a struggle for personhood and validation that looks like a scene in which a couple of 2-year-olds stamp their feet yelling, "Me do it!" and then collapse on the floor in a tantrum.

Clinical Vignette

The transcript excerpt presented in this section is an example of the beginning of a destructive cycle of interaction between parents and child. The argument used by the child is so common that there must be a course in high school called How to Make Your Parents Eat Their Words. Mr. and Mrs. Calden came into treatment with their 13-year-old daughter, Mandy, because she was skipping school, openly defying her parents' directions, and screaming obscenities at them.

The parents entered the room, sat down, and immediately adopted a posture of dejection. Jim Calden was heavy and well dressed. Anne Calden was so thin that she seemed engulfed by her sweat suit. Mandy sat between them with an angry, challenging expression on her face.

A juvenile court probation officer had referred the Caldens to my colleague Barbara Goldstein after Mr. and Mrs. Calden spoke to him about wanting to file an incorrigibility petition on Mandy. The probation officer felt that this was more a case for therapy than court action. Barbara was a 65-year-old therapist who had extensive experience in individual therapies and had begun practicing family therapy in the last few years. Her supportive, motherly nature had served her in good stead through many serious cases during 40 years of clinical practice.

Barbara approached the initial session with the Caldens with her customary smile and good nature. Early in the session Mr. Calden began directing his usual lecture at Mandy: "Everything we tell you not to do, you do it." Since he didn't seem to notice that his wife was crying and wiping at her eyes with a tissue, Barbara commented on Mrs. Calden's behavior in a way that was intended to point out the couple's need to be closer: "I understand. It doesn't give you much of a chance for each other, does it?" Hearing this, Mandy immediately leaned forward in her seat, pointed a finger at her mother, and yelled, "Then send me away! You threatened you'd call an orphanage before, Mom. Why don't you do it again? I'll bet you never told her (*pointing to the therapist*) that."

When the therapist and parents began to close ranks in even this small way, the teenager directed her first assault at her mother. Mrs. Calden already felt like a failure as a parent and felt guilty about the failure. Mandy picked at that guilt and inflamed it by accusing her mother of a crime. She implied that her mother was the cause of the family's problems and her own misbehavior. The therapist, meanwhile, assessed the level of abuse by noticing whether or not the parents responded with credulity to their child's charges. If abusive comments are believed, the child is in greater control.

The following segment of the therapy session demonstrates how Mandy, who leveled accusations against her parents in shrill tones, took control of the interview and succeeded in getting her parents to defend their actions against her charges:

Mrs. Calden, responding to the earlier accusations in a pleading tone of voice, insisted, "I have never called an orphanage."

"Bullshit," replied Mandy.

Her mother continued in her apologetic tone: "You are not an orphan."

"You called a home or something. I was listening on the other phone. That's exactly what you did!"

Mr. Calden tried to speak (for the second time) and was interrupted by Mandy, who continued her loud assault. "That's what started all this!" she yelled.

The childlike nature of the interaction grew, with Mr. Calden finally saying, "That's what you *want* to think."

"You were eavesdropping on my telephone conversations?" Mrs. Calden asked.

Mandy's mother raised a reasonable concern about her daughter's behavior in eavesdropping on a parental phone conversation. Mandy spoke as if her mother had done such a terrible thing by calling about placement that any action on her own part was justified.

Mandy again succeeded in intimidating her mother into dropping her attempt to call her to task for misbehavior. She snarled, "I knew what you were doing."

Mrs. Calden muttered, "Well," but couldn't seem to think of anything else to say.

Mandy continued, "You had it written down and everything."

The best her mother could do in response was, "Then you're mistaken." Mrs. Calden responded defensively to her daughter's accusation and had forgotten about addressing her concerns about Mandy's eavesdropping.

The image of an interaction between 2-year-olds was evoked as Mandy insisted, "No, I'm not!"

"I never called anybody."

"Yes, you did, Mom!"

Mrs. Calden was blowing her nose and wiping her tears as her daughter spoke to her in the angry but composed manner of a mother scolding her errant daughter: "You threatened you were going to take me to juvie. You threatened you were going to call the police. What else are you going to do? Why don't you just send me away, then? I'd rather be anywhere than here."

Mandy again used a powerful technique against parents who felt they'd failed. She steered the conversation further away from the appropriateness of her behavior by accusing her parents of not loving her and wanting to get rid of her.

Mr. Calden attempted to intervene by saying, "You won't have it better with other families." Mandy gave only an exasperated sigh in response, as if she had just heard the town idiot speak.

Mrs. Calden turned to Barbara and said sadly, "I fight with her in the morning to get up."

Mandy replied, "No, you don't."

"I fight with her to get her to go to bed."

"No, you don't."

Mandy was badgering her mother and crippling her ability to speak. Mandy's manner was similar to that of a lawyer who tries to discredit witnesses by confusing them.

Mrs. Calden continued, "It's a fight all the time."

Barbara, hoping to change the mood of the interview and to reestablish Mandy in the role of the identified patient then asked, "When does Mandy go back to school?"

Mrs. Calden replied, "She went back yesterday."

"How did the day go, Mandy?" Barbara asked, turning to the teenager.

Before Mandy could answer Barbara's question, her mother replied, "We don't know. She won't tell us."

Withholding or controlling information is a more advanced method for gaining power over parents. As previously discussed, by acting as if she'd listened in on a phone conversation Mandy verified her mother's intentions. Mandy had gotten information regarding placement, court action, etc.

As Barbara worked with the family and encouraged Mr. Calden to comfort his wife, Mandy withdrew. She sat slumped forward with her face in her hands. Suddenly, Mrs. Calden began to describe her daughter's and husband's interactions to the therapist: "They argue, the two of them. He doesn't stop; she doesn't stop. She's illogical, he's even more illogical. And they just keep at each other."

Mandy had attacked and discredited her mother to the point where Mrs. Calden now began to justify her actions by accusing her husband of mishandling the situation. Even if he had done so, Mandy was still choreographing the present struggle between her parents by attacking her mother. Mrs. Calden now lumped her daughter and husband together as if they were coconspirators. In response, they argued like siblings.

This confusion of proper roles is a course family discussions in therapy often take, a course that further incapacitates parents by putting them at odds with each other. Differences that exist between them become amplified. Although in this case the adolescent was probably trying to surface a serious conflict between her parents, her emotionally abusive way of dealing with the parental struggle amplified the abusive-ness between the parents and made matters worse. As we shall see, Mandy verified this interpretation of her behavior: She revealed her concern for her parents' relationship by offering to leave the room when Barbara began discussing the relationship between her parents.

Barbara asked Mrs. Calden about her husband's behavior: "Is he illogical with you?"

"Generally. It's hard to follow how he's thinking."

Barbara continued, "How is Jim illogical with you?"

Mandy interrupted, "Hey, can I go out and wait? Please?"

Without responding to Mandy, Barbara encouraged Mrs. Calden, and she continued, "His thoughts are hard to follow. He says things that don't have anything to do with what's going on. The hardest part is to sit and listen to him argue with Mandy because she catches him like that (*snaps her fingers*)."

Barbara addressed Mr. Calden, "Are you as upset with this as Anne is?"

He answered halfheartedly, "Uh-huh."

"With this arguing?" Barbara prompted.

Mr. Calden replied, "Any little thing, like a pin dropped, and I get very upset."

Mandy once again inserted herself between her parents by verbally abusing them, and Mr. and Mrs. Calden once again took the bait, demonstrating that a recursive cycle had developed, with Mandy's abusiveness increasing the conflict between her parents, and her parents' accusations toward each other increasing Mandy's abusiveness.

Later in the session Mr. Calden surprised Barbara by showing a more compassionate side of himself by saying, "I'm very worried that Mandy might do something to hurt herself."

Mandy responded, "If you guys would just leave me alone!"

Mr. Calden continued, "We had a lot of problems back then. We just let you go."

Mandy retorted, "No, you didn't. It all started when you started calling places. When I thought that I wasn't worth anything, that's when all this started. Everything was fine before then."

This is an example of the ease with which an adolescent can resort to psychological abuse. Here Mandy claimed that her self-esteem had been crushed by her parents. She was implying that her parents' attempts to get treatment for her so devastated her feelings about herself that her behavioral problems were completely their fault.

Mr. Calden stuck to the subject of Mandy's behavior by saying to her, "I don't think it was fine. You had a whole list of things you were doing that weren't right."

Mandy again attempted to determine the course of the conversation by redirecting it away from the topic of her behavior: "Dad, you're talking about something I wasn't even talking about, again."

Conclusion

The foregoing transcript excerpt demonstrates the course interviews often take when parents feel battered emotionally by a child. It's often difficult to tell whether the parents' conflict and depression is bringing about the child's abusiveness or if the child's abusiveness is bringing about the parents' conflict and depression. In either case, the cycle spells disaster; it has the quality of a satellite's decaying orbit in space, the altitude slowly dropping until the satellite hits the atmosphere, bursts into flames, and falls to earth as a cinder.

CHILD PROTECTIVE SERVICES: THE HAMMER OF THE '90s

There's a serious need in our society for a system that sees to it that children are protected from abuse. As is typical of our society—and perhaps of human nature—the pendulum has been allowed to swing from one extreme to the other. Thirty years ago there were few programs to adequately protect children from the abusive whims of parents. Parental rights seemed inviolate. Now, in the 1980s and '90s, rapid action is taken in response to reports of suspected child abuse and neglect. Child protection laws have expedited the removal of children from their homes. The difficulty comes when society tries to protect children without violating the rights of parents.

The courts now regularly neglect parents' rights in order to ensure that children are safe. Children are removed on the report of a single caseworker, and the rules of evidence often don't apply. This shift in societal attitude, away from the rights of parents and toward those of children, has unwittingly offered newfound power to children who may not use that power wisely. A common method for abusing this power is seen when children threaten to call child protective services in order to incapacitate their parents. Some children have the audacity to call and falsely report abuse to police or teachers.

A classic example of how devastating the use of child protective services power can be is demonstrated by the Markman family. When their daughter, Samantha, was 10 years old, she went to school and made an innocuous statement to a teacher that implied she'd been physically abused. In fact, there had been no abuse. The school, without contacting the parents to clarify the situation, contacted child protective services. The caseworker who was sent to the Markmans' house was a new worker in her early 20s who was accusatory toward Mr. and Mrs. Markman despite the absence of evidence of abuse. The Markmans' attorney told Mr. and Mrs. Markman that if they responded angrily to a child protective services worker, they would look guilty. Therefore, they cooperated and went along with the humiliation of being lectured on what they could and couldn't do with their children. The department of social services soon decided to close the Markman case as unsubstantiated, although the Markmans were registered in a national database as a couple who had been suspected of child abuse. Six months after the experience with child protective services, Mr. Markman was wrestling with his son and daughter. He had Samantha in a benign wrestling hold and she asked to be released. Mr. Markman responded by saying that she had to say, "I give up" before he'd let her up. Samantha replied that if he didn't let her up, she'd go to school and tell the counselor that he'd touched her "privates." Upon hearing this remark, the devastated father went to his bedroom and cried for 30 minutes. At the time the Markmans entered therapy 4 years later, Mr. Markman hadn't touched, kissed, or hugged Samantha in 4 years. His response of anger and fear had more to do with the abuse he had been subjected to at the hands of child protective services than with Samantha's impulsive comment. Her threat wouldn't have meant much if her father hadn't already been falsely accused of wrongdoing and mistreated as a result.

It continues to be difficult to figure out how to protect children without mistreating parents and wrongly breaking up families. The justice system has always believed it's better to let ten guilty people go free than to punish one who's innocent. However, this philosophy is more difficult to live by when it's stated as follows: It's better to let ten abused children remain in the home rather than break up one innocent family.

There are some obvious problems with the manner in which child protection is carried out. Any experienced attorney will advise parents to do exactly what the caseworker says, because parents have few rights. In a courtroom a person is innocent until proven guilty; in child protection cases parents are guilty until proven innocent. The burden of proof is on the suspects. Overzealous social workers may remove children from their homes on the basis of hearsay and innuendo. Even when substantial evidence is clearly lacking, the children may be kept in custody and an investigation is held to justify continued placement. Caseworkers may interview friends, relatives, and acquaintances with the specific intent of proving that the removal of the children was not a mistake.

Even in substantiated cases where removal of children is justified, there's a major discrepancy between public policy and parental rights. The latter are often so neglected that parents who've mishandled their children are publicly humiliated and consequently withdraw from the situation and from their children. These parents are then even less likely to do what's needed to get their children back. The most unjust element of parental abuse by the system can be seen in the guidelines parents must meet to get their children returned after they've been removed. It isn't enough for parents to correct their mistakes. They're often expected to meet standards for parenthood that far exceed those required for the protection of the child. In fact, in order to keep their children they must exceed standards that parents in general aren't expected to even meet.

A good example of standards being imposed beyond those required for protection of the children is the case of the Henderson family. Mary was a single parent who used poor judgment and lived for a year with a man who'd been undressing and fondling her 8-year-old daughter. Mary learned of the abuse when her daughter told a teacher, who then called Mary and child protective services. A caseworker came out the same day and removed the 8-year-old, Julie, as well as Mark, 2, and Joey, 5. Mary reacted quickly to the allegation that Julie was being molested: Once she discussed the molestation with Julie and was convinced that her account of the fondling was true, Mary insisted that her boyfriend move out of the house immediately and refrained from further contact with him. Despite the fact that the perpe-

trator was removed from contact with them, Mary's children, weren't
returned home. They were being punished, and their human rights were
violated by their removal from a home their mother had made safe for them.
Although therapy for Mary and her children was a reasonable requirement,
the family remained separated until Mary had completed a lengthy individual therapy process and her therapist was convinced that she'd resolved
issues that were perhaps related to the sexual abuse.

Mary's story is a classic case of blaming the victim. In addition to
being required to have therapy, Mary was criticized by the caseworker for
clutter in her house and for her failure to make the beds. The caseworker
also asked her embarrassing and intrusive questions about her sexual
partners and the kinds of sexual acts she engaged in. The foster care
worker told Mary she had to have a house that had a separate bedroom
for each of the children before they could be returned. One year after the
removal of her children, Mary still did not have them back. Her chances
of getting them back dropped even further when she became so discouraged with the demands and humiliation that she became lethargic and
depressed. She stopped keeping regular visitation appointments with the
children and would no longer respond civilly to the caseworker. Mary had
become so discouraged that she yelled at the caseworker in court; this
behavior proved to the court and to the caseworker that she was indeed
an unfit parent.

In cases of unsubstantiated abuse, parents are often required to take
parenting classes and meet several requirements before the case can be
closed—despite the fact that there was insufficient evidence to prove
abuse. Parents may be threatened and harassed, and they have no legal
recourse at all. If parents take any legal action, the court often retaliates
against them. Retaliation may be directed not only against parents but
also, at times, against the caseworker. When a child who has been
returned home is later injured, the error is often blamed on the caseworker. In other words, caseworkers who are willing to take a risk to help
parents reunite with their children are often penalized. Many have been
fired or scapegoated on the front page of the newspaper when additional
molestation of a child is made public. It's no wonder that many caseworkers feel they must err on the side of caution no matter what the consequences to the family.

The aggressiveness with which laws have been aimed at punishing
parents has changed the complexion of family life and child protection.
Samantha Markman only wanted her way in a wrestling match and was
appalled that she'd alienated her father. Other young people may not be
so benevolent and can actually force their parents into submission with
threatened or actual reports of child abuse. Such reports lead to a situation
in which the system helps young people abuse their parents. Such abuse

occurred when 14-year-old Rebecca started dating older boys and high school dropouts—it was almost as though her partners were picked primarily to worry her mother. Knowing that her mother had had a great many sexual exploits as a teenager and had used drugs, Rebecca found a way to stop her mother from setting limits on how late she stayed out with her boyfriends. One day when her mother tried to ground her, Rebecca proclaimed, "Fine, then I'll just go sleep with the drug dealers in Detroit and tell everyone that you kicked me out." Rebecca's mother became so panic-stricken that she dropped any attempt to control the girl. Rebecca's proclamation was particularly effective: In a single sentence she accused her mother of neglect and threatened to use drugs, engage in sexual activity, run away, and court infection with AIDS.

Power was also wielded by 15-year-old Harold, who upon hearing his parents issue restrictions would begin to moan that life was hopeless and that there was no point in going on. Harold would accuse his parents of abusing him by keeping him locked up in the house against his will. He said they were no better than the parents in Michigan who had their 10-year-old daughter chained to her urine-soaked bed every night. Though such an accusation may seem ludicrous to some readers, it's amazing how seriously many parents take such statements from their children; they hear them as an honest commentary on how horrible they are as parents.

Teenagers eventually discover that they have real power. The moment they discover this power they must decide whether they will confine it to minor misbehavior and mild threats or expand it into a pattern of more serious abuse.

EMOTIONAL TERRORISM AS ABUSE

Webster's New World Dictionary, Third College Edition, defines terrorism as "The act of terrorizing; use of force or threats to demoralize, intimidate, and subjugate, esp. such use as a political weapon or policy; the demoralization and intimidation produced in this way." For our purposes the concept of emotional terrorism will be used to describe certain methods of revolt that young people use when their parents are requiring them to do things they aren't pleased with. Young people use emotional terrorism which plays on their parents' fear and guilt, when they threaten to harm themselves if their parents don't give in to their demands. Even 6-year-olds use emotional terrorism—when, for example, they threaten to run away because their parents are so "mean" or threaten to hold their breath until they "turn blue and die." These simple yet powerful threats become progressively more sophisticated and threatening as children grow older.

When one mother said no to her teenage son the boy replied, "Satan told me you would say that." If a parent demands that a child stop skipping school and threatens to accompany him or her to class to make sure the child gets there, the response might be, "Then I'll just quit school, and it will be your fault." If a parent tells a daughter that she can't associate with a certain boy, she may threaten, "Then I'll just run away with him." If a parent opposes a girl's sexual activity, she may respond, "I'll just get pregnant then." In more extreme forms of emotional terrorism, young people will blame thoughts of suicide or minor acts of self-abuse on their parents' attempts to influence their choice of friends. When told that they may not do what they want, some adolescents have said that they "can't go on" if parents don't reverse their decision.

What position should therapists take when they must tell parents what to do with children who are threatening themselves? Therapists themselves may be frightened by the young person's threat. The guidelines used for dealing with political terrorism also hold true for emotional terrorism. Almost all governments clearly say (despite some covert attempts to do otherwise), "We never negotiate with terrorists." As with any manipulative behavior, if terrorism succeeds, it will be repeated. If terrorists' demands are met when they take hostages, they are more likely to take hostages again the next time there's a problem (terrorists may, of course, use even more extreme tactics to get the desired response). The risk of repetition is the same with emotional terrorism. A therapist who thinks the position of the parents is reasonable should advise them to hold that position despite threats from the child. Helping parents maintain their position is difficult for the therapist when the parents are discouraged and certain that their offspring is the one who won't submit to authority, no matter how powerfully or firmly it is presented. This point in the interview is when the therapist learns what the parents' deepest fears are. The therapist must draw on his or her years of experience to assure the parents that children much more rebellious than theirs have responded to intervention. Desperate parents may ask the therapist, "What would you do if this were your child?" The therapist can respond, "I hope I would put aside my fears, although I know that wouldn't be easy, and give my child the guidance and strength he or she is crying out for."

If a threat of suicide has been made, the therapist should tell the parents that it's time to find out once and for all if their child is disturbed enough to carry out such a threat. If parents honestly believe their teen might attempt suicide, they must be directed to put the young person on 24-hour supervision with a mandate that he or she not be left alone for a moment. Arranging a suicide watch is often difficult; parents claim that no one can stay home with the teen and that the family is alone in the world. The therapist must believe that help is available and must spend as much time as is necessary to identify helpers in the family, at school, in church, and in the community. A suicide watch may be just the sign of love and commitment from a parent that a depressed young person needs. Conversely, if a parent is covertly supporting the acting out, that parent gets inconvenienced until the suicide threat has passed. Many parents see reason in the argument that action must be taken while their child is still a minor and they can intervene using the courts, hospitalization, treatment programs, and special schools. If parents wait until the child becomes an adult, when these options are no longer available, their child could wind up dead or in prison.

Once an adolescent begins to respond to parental strength, as most do, parents can begin to work out ways to grant some of the freedoms and rights their child has been asking for. If a teenager carries out damaging or self-destructive actions in order to stop the parents from taking control, the therapist can help the parents plan countermaneuvers. If a teenager is truly in danger, the therapist will encourage the parents to take more decisive remedial action (see Chapter 6 on assessment and intervention).

When faced with the need to help parents take action, therapists must decide whether to be directive or nondirective. Join me on a journey through a mythical land where the question of whether to be directive or nondirective is discussed 24 hours a day. In lands constructed of fantasy, everyday activities may be approached in unexpected ways. In Ray Bradbury's futuristic novel *Farenheit 451*, all books were outlawed and firemen existed for the purpose of seeking out and burning contraband books. In our mythical land therapists exist to help people in distress avoid painful change. The only approach clinicians are allowed to practice is *status quo therapy*. Regardless of the intensity of a person's pain, status quo therapists must help clients learn to live with that pain and all of the accompanying problems.

As a professional, you will start reading about this notion of status quo therapy and will immediately say, "But that's not what therapists were put here to do. We were trained to help people change their lives and find new creative solutions to problems." As you read the following description of status quo therapy, you may be struck by how closely the techniques therapists use in this fantasy world resemble methods commonly used in our own world. I suspect the resemblance isn't a coincidence. The discussion of status quo therapy may lead to more clues toward understanding why adolescents become abusive and why therapy often doesn't succeed in helping them and their families.

Directive versus Nondirective Approaches

How to Maintain the Status Quo Without Really Trying

The debate over the virtues of directive versus nondirective therapies has been going on since Freud first advised therapists to sit back and wait for things to unfold. The directive therapist is thought of as controlling and heartless, the nondirective therapist as ineffectual and passive. An area of expertise is now emerging that can heal many of the conflicts between clinical orientations. Any school of thought has an equal opportunity to excel in the development of skills used for maintaining the status quo in families.

Through the ages the helping professions have flourished out of a strong desire to reduce the pain and suffering of the human condition. A wide range of professionals expend an extraordinary amount of energy attempting to help individual clients and families in need. One particular brand of intervention—*status quo therapy*—puts the client's comfort before all else. Not only are all schools of thought represented in this approach, but its practice typically results in dedicated clients as well as respect from the community.

The practice of status quo therapy is performed by therapists who blindly trust their unconscious to keep them on track. However, the time has come for this field to follow the example of professional approaches that have preceded it.

As was the case with Ericksonian hypnotherapy, strategic therapy, psychoanalysis, and many other schools of thought, a conceptual framework must be developed for those skills that have typically been seen as inborn and spontaneous. By understanding what underlies the success of this approach, future therapists will be able to learn the skills required and those with an innate talent in this direction may hone their mastery of what is a complex procedure. More and more, authors in the therapy field are now recognizing the importance of status quo therapy. Jay Haley (1980) has regularly referred to the creative methods employed for stabilizing unstable family systems. Joel Bergman (1985) has pointed out a number of techniques that, if properly used, will dramatically increase a therapist's effectiveness in helping people avoid change by maintaining the status quo. What follows here is an account that will help the reader differentiate status quo therapy from those insensitive, calculating approaches that use directives and redefinitions to bring about uncomfortable or frightening changes in the very fabric of a client's existence.

Now that we know how the practice of status quo therapy emerged, we must begin with a clear definition of it. This therapy, which is used to provide stability, can best be described as *any mode of treatment in which the therapist, actively or passively, responds to an individual or family in such a manner that comfort is assured. Undue distress, above and beyond that normally experienced by the client or family, is carefully detoured and more frightening crises are averted by keeping the therapy consistent with the client's or family's view of reality.*

Let us now explore the benefits of such an approach for the client and guidelines for its proper application.

BENEFITS FOR THE CLIENT

Clients routinely approach therapists covertly requesting the status quo therapy approach. People in therapy often resist the therapist's suggestions when they're pushed to change how they do things. It seems safe to assume, then, that status quo therapy would be the treatment of choice for most clients. It must hold significant advantages for it to be so widely requested. The most obvious of these advantages is that gratification of the client's primary needs is maintained. A client who feels unloved can find a place to feel accepted. Those in distress find a place where a caring person is available on short notice to help them resolve their crisis—regardless of how many times the crisis is repeated or how long it lasts.

Almost as impressive as the maintenance of need gratification for the client is the importance this approach places on avoiding inconvenience to significant others. This avoidance of inconvenience is particularly clear when an adolescent is being treated individually. Treating the teenager in isolation spares the parents needless stress and energy. For treatment to proceed properly, the therapist must withhold from the parents details of treatment that could result in their becoming distressed and having to take action. In this way a serious family crisis can be averted and the adolescent can remain the sole focus of attention. Another example of the avoidance of inconvenience to significant others exists in marital therapy when one spouse is seen alone. To treat the individual properly, the therapist must demonstrate sympathy for his or her distress in the relationship and must meet those emotional needs that the spouse is no longer attending to. In this way the distressed spouse becomes calm and no longer feels an urgent need for change in the relationship; this placidity may last for several years. If the therapist fails to keep the client calm, the couple will still be helped in the long run: The odds then increase dramatically that the couple will wind up divorced and be permanently freed from having to put up with each other (Gurman & Kniskern, 1991).

In each of the above examples the therapist helps reestablish and support the status quo. The client is pleased because he or she feels better, and those close to the client feel less pressure to change. This discussion of comfort leads nicely into an exploration of the advantages this approach holds for the profession of psychotherapy as a whole.

BENEFITS FOR THE PROFESSION

Foremost among the benefits for the profession of status quo therapy is the positive effect this approach has on the public's image of the psychotherapy profession. Since clients receiving status quo therapy come to depend heavily upon their therapists, it's always clear that whatever change occurs is solely the result of the therapy. Friends, relatives, and community agents refer numerous new cases and speak highly of the profession, because clients attribute their improvement entirely to their therapist. Status quo therapy's positive influence is further dramatized by the fact that clients usually feel worse whenever they take a break from treatment. Friends and relatives then make comments like, "I told you you shouldn't have stopped your sessions!" Therapists can then explain relapses as the result of "resistance" rather than as any failing on their part. This tendency to attribute clients' improvement to the therapist but to deny any responsibility on the part of the therapist for relapse in clients further ensures that the clients won't make the serious mistake of assuming they alone are responsible for improvement. It's well known that such false confidence only leads to disappointing relapses, anyway.

This discussion leads the reader to the next logical conclusion regarding advantages for the profession: Clients responding properly to status quo therapy come in frequently for sessions, rarely cancel or fail to show up for an appointment, and remain in therapy for extended periods of time. This attendance record assures therapists in private practice a secure income for providing the service requested by the client. A consistent clientele demonstrates the need for therapy in a dramatic way. For community agencies, such an attendance record will satisfy funding sources' growing demands for more direct (face-to-face) contact with clients.

Finally, status quo therapy can resolve another serious problem faced by the therapy profession: The danger exists that if all important family members were included in sessions, these troubled relationships would play themselves out in the therapist's office. This uncomfortable situation can be avoided by the use of techniques that stabilize the crisis and reduce the immediate symptoms *and* that do so without involving people whose presence would endanger the therapist's control of the process. Allowing uncertainties is risky to the reputation of therapy in general as well as to that of the individual therapist.

Readers might conclude that any approach with such advantages is too good to be true. One might also fear that status quo therapy is too specialized a skill to be assimilated. However, the guidelines that follow should put status quo therapy within the reach of any therapist.

TECHNIQUES FOR MAINTAINING THE STATUS QUO

Before one learns the techniques involved, it must be understood that this approach, like many others, can only be taught within limits. Descriptions of possible techniques are intended to open one's mind to a new way of thinking and tap into one's creativity. Because every client or family is different, the therapist must be able to design interventions for that particular system. What follows is a brief, and by no means exhaustive, listing of guidelines for maintaining the status quo.

First and foremost is the importance of making the proper choice of a client or family with whom to implement this approach. One must look for certain characteristics that designate a particular client or family as a "target case." These characteristics can be identified by the therapist's intuitive and intellectual responses to the initial phone call or intake interview. The more amenable case will be one that bears some resemblance to the therapist's own family. This resemblance can be to the therapist's current nuclear family or the family of origin. Obvious structural similarities may become clear as one objectively explores the nature of the client's concerns. The following questions should be considered when choosing a case:

1. Is this individual or family in the same stage of the family life cycle as the therapist (e.g., the run-ragged-by-the-crumb-snatchers stage, the bankrupt-by-college-tuition stage, or the yours-mine-and-ours stage)?
2. Do any of the client's struggles resemble those the therapist has experienced or is currently experiencing (e.g., nagging the drunk to quit lying around and get a decent job—just as the therapist will be doing at home tonight)?
3. Are family members' roles or an individual's interpersonal style reminiscent of the therapist's past relationships (e.g., a small voice in the therapist's head says, "You're an awful lot like my mother and father. I guess that's why I dislike you so much")?

If any of these intellectually based considerations holds true, it can become the basis for effective stabilization of the family using status quo therapy.

There are also intuitive considerations that may offer clues to making a wise choice of the right family or individual in need of stabilization. To identify these factors the therapist must observe his or her spontaneous emotional responses. The following questions may be helpful.

1. Is the therapist having a strong emotional reaction of any kind (e.g., anger, sympathy, pain, or maternal or paternal feelings)?
2. Does the therapist feel an overwhelming responsibility to solve the family's problems (e.g., are the white charger and shining armor coming out of the closet?)?
3. Does the therapist find him- or herself trying to convince the client to become involved or stay involved in therapy (e.g., begging, threatening, or guilt-tripping clients with threats of psychotic breaks if they leave therapy)?
4. Does the therapist find him- or herself inclined to routinely do as the client requests? (e.g., "I want you to see my daughter alone!"—to which the therapist internally responds, "Yes, dear")?

The greater the number of positive responses to these questions, the more likely the therapist's own family is being recreated in some way. The clinician is likely to misread his or her own responses and to label those reactions as proper clinical judgment. In fact, the client system is communicating its fears and perceptions, to which most any therapist would be likely to respond with status-quo-maintaining interventions. Thus, since whatever the family is feeling can be accommodated, the scene is set for ongoing stability.

With the professional system responding strongly to the above influences, a range of specific interventions will be required. Here are some guidelines for helping a client maintain the status quo once an appropriate individual or family is chosen:

- See the individual only, especially if others are obviously involved.
- Encourage the identified patient's involvement in as many treatment systems as possible. After all, more is better.
- Encourage ongoing use of stabilizing psychiatric medications as the first approach to a problem.
- Keep a personal investment in what you feel is best for the client, in spite of evidence to the contrary.
- Encourage lengthy involved discussions about the client's feelings but without directing change.
- Form a coalition with an adolescent to criticize the parents' misbehaviors, and lecture the parents.
- Assume the apparent victim in a marital conflict is truly a victim, and work to rescue him or her.
- Take a stand against another professional involved in the case in such a way that the conflict in the family is replayed among the professionals.
- Become the one person who can keep a suicidal person from killing him- or herself.
- Define a crisis by the client's perception of a crisis, and respond immediately.
- Change the subject when topics discussed begin to arouse conflict.
- Agree to keep a secret with one member of a family, and guarantee general secrecy from everyone else involved.
- Consider clients to be future friends.
- Lend the client money or extend credit on fees.
- Avoid use of a consultant who may encourage interventions that could bring about serious discomfort and change.
- And above all: Never do anything that might upset clients or make them love you less.

Though not complete, these guidelines begin to form an approach toward interventions that will encourage client comfort and stability. This stability may take the form of (1) true complacency on the client's part or (2) serious distress that's familiar, long-standing, and secure. The right choice of client and the judicious use of the techniques discussed create a momentum that will help ensure the outcome that clients seem to desire.

In the naive world of status quo therapy, clients who appear to want to remain unchanged can get therapy that helps them do just that. In reality, however, even adolescents who tell everyone to leave them alone must be seen as people who want things to feel better for themselves and their families.

THREE

Early Warning Signs of Aggression

Overreacting to Aggression in Preteenage Children

B efore therapists begin the treatment of aggression and violence in young children, they must understand how to conceptualize families and children, as well as their problems. In the late 19th and early 20th centuries, as Freudians and neo-Freudians were busy establishing the early psychiatric community, our culture was still caught up in a Victorian view of childhood. Children were viewed as miniature adults, and separate rules and concepts about their growth and development were rare. They were dressed as small adults and were expected to behave like a "little man" or a "young lady." They were "analyzed" with the aid of the same rules, understandings, and diagnoses used for assessing adults; therapists helped children develop insight into their problems and encouraged them to express their feelings in words.

In the era after the world wars, society began moving toward a benevolent, indulgent view that emphasized the importance of play in childhood and granted children the freedom to grow as individuals. School programs were organized around enlightened views of early childhood development, and the teenage years were understood as a transitional period between childhood and adulthood. Now, in the mid-1990s, both society and the field of psychotherapy are swinging back toward a new form of the "little man" conceptualization of children. Despite liberal child-rearing techniques, children are once again being treated like miniature adults. The last two or three generations of children have grown up with adult worries and fears—fears based on facts. Whereas the young adults of today grew up in fear of a nuclear holocaust, children now live in fear of acid rain, destruction of the ozone layer, damage to the environment, crime running rampant, and death from AIDS. They're taught negotiation skills and methods for thwarting attackers at 4 or 5 years of age. No wonder preteenagers and teenagers are becoming insistent about being able to run their own lives and make decisions for themselves! They are expected to perform adult functions years earlier than their parents and grandparents were expected to.

In view of the precocity of today's children, it follows that 10-year-olds are being labeled with adult diagnoses such as explosive personality disorder and schizophrenia. Then those children are given adult treatment as if their families didn't exist. Young children of 7 or 8 are being hospitalized for extended periods of psychiatric and residential treatment to resolve their feelings, and they're medicated with adult antidepressant and antipsychotic medications when aggression is the presenting symptom. This tendency to diagnose disorders and mental illness in children has a way of locking in everyone's understanding of a child's behavior. The children come to understand themselves as damaged people who aren't in control of themselves. Parents become confused and don't know whether to push or pamper their handicapped offspring; they are given new understandings of their children that define the children they love as aliens they can no longer recognize.

When children look into their parents' eyes, they see reflections of themselves, and those parental reflections tell children who they are. For instance, a 1-year-old boy who toddles along on stiff, shaky legs, having just discovered how to balance himself, has a big grin on his face because the adults are so proud of him. As he walks across the hardwood floor of the family room to explore, he suddenly loses his balance, falls forward, and hits his head and elbow on the floor. He knows it hurts, but he isn't sure how to react. He looks at the nearest adult to see how badly he's hurt. If his father looks terrified and shouts, "Oh my God!" as he runs toward the boy, the child knows he was really hurt and bursts into tears. If that same father, seeing that there isn't a serious injury, calmly says, "That's okay, honey, you're all right; go get your train," the boy knows he's all right, dusts himself off, and goes on walking.

Consider a 5-year-old boy who can't seem to stop his temper tantrums. He throws himself on the ground, kicking and screaming; sometimes kicks adults; and attacks other kids and hits them with toys. When he looks in his parents' eyes to see if he's okay, does he see a little boy having a tantrum or a psychiatrically disturbed monster who can't be understood? Does he see fear and helplessness or a reasonable level of concern? When adults overreact to children's symptoms with diagnoses and hospitalizations, children learn from their reflection in the eyes of parents and therapists, who they are now and what they're going to become. Children either identify themselves as sick or believe themselves to be normal people with problems that can be solved. If their reflection is of a disordered person, they are less likely to get better and exhibit more normal behavior. When a preschooler with a disturbed identity reaches adolescence, the seed of disturbance that was planted early in life has a high risk of germinating into full-blown aggression.

TYPICAL MISDIAGNOSES

To understand why children are being diagnosed and treated as sick, let's look at some presentations of problems in young children and the diagnoses they might inspire:

♦ Christina, age 3, was brought to therapy because she was stealing things from stores like gum and small toys, while her mother shopped. In addition, Christina had been walking up to men at their apartment's swimming pool and grabbing their genitals. Could this 3-year-old have become sexually deviant? Had she developed a budding character disorder in her short life? Could she be suffering from repressed anger as the result of her parents' recent divorce?

♦ James, age 8, was taken by his father to a clinical psychologist for evaluation after he became sullen, withdrawn, and apparently angry. His father felt James's anger was caused by repressed feelings that had accumulated as the result of rejection by his mother (now a noncustodial parent). In the evaluation interview, James was playing with a toy space shuttle. The psychologist told James that a woman had died on the space shuttle and asked him which woman he would like to see dead. The little boy, knowing what was expected of him, said he wanted his mother to die. The psychologist proceeded to testify in court that James's mother had done irreparable damage to him and should never be allowed to see him again. Could this 8-year-old boy be clinically depressed? Could his "pathological" hatred of his mother have come to overshadow the bond they'd shared for many years so that he no longer loved her at all? Could this be a case for antidepressant medication?

♦ Ethan, age 6, was brought to therapy because his mother reported him "violently assaulting" his 2-year-old sister, Sarah. He hit and pushed her every chance he got. His mother, an experienced and educated parent, had tried everything she could think of. She had used time-outs and behavioral charts with rewards, and she had tried ignoring the problem, but Ethan continued to push and punch Sarah. Could Ethan's situation be a case where long-term play therapy is in order to get at the roots of his deep-seated hostility? Might inpatient hospitalization be necessary, considering the danger this boy represents, so that experts can explore his hostility on a daily basis?

Although these children were displaying serious symptoms that had to be addressed, it was the clinical orientation of the therapist that determined which of the many available treatment methods would be used. Are these children's symptoms manifestations of psychopathology, or might their difficulties be telling us metaphorically what's upsetting them? Might these children be providing clues for understanding their difficulty with someone who is a central figure in their lives? Might the children be spontaneously manifesting what is subtly communicated to them? Could these children be little beacons showing us what in the here-and-now needs to be addressed?

In Christina's case I explored the possibility that she might be a victim of sexual abuse and concluded that she wasn't being molested. I learned that her mother was bitter about how Christina's father had handled their divorce and that her mother's anger at men, seething just beneath the surface of her daughter's behavior, was revealing itself in destructive ways. For example, Christina's mother picked up married men in bars. If they had sex with her, she took this as proof that men are loathsome creatures; if they wouldn't have sex with her, she felt rejected and criticized them bitterly. Christina's actions around the pool could certainly be a message about her mother's sexually expressed anger at men. Such anger can be resolved in the present. As for the child's stealing: I learned later that Christina's mother had been having a year-long affair with her best friend's husband. Christina's behavior could be understood as a metaphor for her mother's stealing her friend's mate. I asked Christina's mother to look at her own lifestyle and make decisions about what kind of example she wanted to set for her daughter. Once the mother began changing how she handled her anger at men, the preschooler's symptoms disappeared. If Christina had been labeled a budding young thief, she might well have grown into a teenager who shoplifts regularly.

The emotional paralysis that James was experiencing was easily explained: His withdrawal from emotional expression was the only reasonable action he could take when caught in the hostilities between the two people he loved most in the world. By not expressing anything, James was avoiding siding with one parent against the other. When the case was heard in court to decide whether his mother should be removed from James's life, the judge recognized the symptoms of a divorce war and ordered increased visitation with James by his mother, provided mother and son work with a therapist to help improve their relationship. When the relationship between the parents was mediated by a therapist, James gradually began making friends and pulling out of his "depression." If James's response to his parents' difficulties had been left untreated or misunderstood as a genetically inherited predisposition, he could easily have become one of those youngsters who are in and out of therapy throughout childhood and adolescence.

In trying to discover the source of Ethan's hostility toward his little sister, I learned that the 6-year-old, his sister, and his mother had recently moved into a new home, which the family had to share with a house-mate. I assigned a time each evening for Ethan's mother to encourage him to use a foam baseball bat to beat on a pillow (as a replacement for his sister). By ritualizing the boy's misbehavior and encouraging his mother to allow him to express anger in a safe way, I was able to decrease Ethan's aggressiveness toward his sister. As he improved, Ethan began screaming at the family's housemate without any apparent provocation. Ethan's mother overheard her housemate making shame-inducing comments to Ethan about his behavior. For example, she told him that he was a "bad boy" and that he was hurting his mother. Such negativity was so foreign to him that he became confused and upset. Once Ethan's mother became aware of this provocation, it was a straightforward task for her to discuss the housemate's intervention with her and to set up ground rules. The housemate became angry and defensive, and the family eventually moved elsewhere. Once the housemate was confronted, Ethan stopped his aggressive behavior within a few weeks. If he'd been labeled as characterological or dangerous, Ethan might have become a dangerous teenager.

Any of these three children could have been hospitalized, drugged, and subjected to therapy over a long period of time. They would have begun to develop an identity as a psychiatric patient. Their parents, who only needed to solve a problem they were having trouble understanding, might have suffered the pain and stigma of having a child branded as abnormal because constant psychiatric care was required. In many such situations, parents and children only need a nudge in the right direction. It's remarkable how many cases in treatment are ones in which the severity of a problem has been caused by people or agencies who interfere with a natural healing process and usurp the role of parent. Often the damage comes after parents are removed from therapeutic leadership of their family. When parents are disenfranchised, young children (as well as teenagers) also suffer. When experts usurp the role of parent and disregard the family as the primary healing element for children, the process becomes inhumane. Instead of packaging and labeling children as if they were aliens from outer space, professionals must help parents do the tough and tender job of loving and controlling their children. No matter how kindly the professional, the process must promote healing as well.

The key to seeing a preteenage problem in a therapeutic way is to expand the therapist's view of who's involved in the problem and focus on the people already in the child's life. When there's a struggle going on between two people, there's usually a third person involved (Haley, 1976; Price, 1988). Even when one person seems to be a solitary violent perpetrator, it's wise to look for two other people who are embroiled in the drama.

COMMON SYMPTOMS AND THEIR MESSAGES

What are the most common aggressive symptoms in children aged 12 and under, and what are those symptoms telling us metaphorically about the concerns in children's lives? Metaphorical aggressive symptoms are typically symptoms that are either violent in nature, threaten violence, or allude to devastation due to violence.

♦ Whenever a child acts out violently, the wise therapist tries to understand the covert theme. A girl who hits her mother with toys and other objects might be signaling the upset she feels over incidents in which her father hits her mother. A small boy who beats his head against a wall might be trying to tell the therapist how upset he is that his mother flies into a terrifying rage when she's angry.

♦ Violent metaphorical content is also present when children verbally threaten bodily harm. A girl who screams, "I'm going to kill you!" at her mother could be pointing out that her father is so angry with her grandmother that he'd like to kill her. A young boy raising a knife to his mother might be demonstrating his father's rage over the divorce the father didn't want; the boy's father may even be subtly influencing his son to retaliate for him against his ex-wife.

♦ Self-destructive threats, suicide attempts, or statements about not wanting to live—all these may allude to violence or the threat of violence that exists among those a child loves. Many young children say, "I wish I were dead," when it is the parent who is depressed and feels unable to go on; such children could be telling us, for example, that a parent is drinking him- or herself to death.

♦ Children who stop taking care of themselves may be signaling a threatening situation. For example, a girl who stops washing, eating, or exercising may be indicating that someone around her wants to give up on life; perhaps her father hasn't recovered from the death of her mother and only goes on because his daughter needs him. The same symptom may point out that a grandfather, who had a stroke recently, can't decide whether life is worth enduring and is considering suicide. A boy I treated called his school and made a bomb threat after his mother was diagnosed with cancer.

♦ Sexually aggressive acting out (not including mutual and consensual experimentation) toward other children or adults can be interpreted metaphorically. Such is the case when a child, often very young, forcefully touches adults' breasts or genitalia without apparent provocation. Someone might be touching the child inappropriately, but there are often explanations other than sexual abuse of the child; an automatic assumption of sexual abuse may be a hasty one. There may, for example, be a struggle between the child's parents where one parent wants to have sex and the other withholds it as a way of wielding power.

♦ Fears, fantasies, or delusions of physical or sexual assault that are experienced by young children can also be viewed as metaphorical in nature. A child's repeated nightmare of burglars could be telling us of her mother's fear of someone breaking into the house and raping the mother (perhaps because of an actual rape in the past). A young boy who uses a lot of black crayon to draw pictures of people shooting and stabbing others could have an older brother who's involved with drug dealers, and he may be expressing a fear for his older brother's life.

Thus, symptoms with violent content must be viewed as possible attempts on the child's part to convey information about a situation metaphorically. There's no one metaphorical message attached to any particular symptom, yet experience suggests some general areas for the therapist to explore when faced with such symptoms in preteenagers. A therapist must take the risk of seeing symptoms in new and unique ways. Rigid views that assume psychopathology have become archaic. If we think in metaphors and messages, we need only pay attention to what children are telling us by their actions, rather than their words, and then ask ourselves why they're choosing particular actions at particular times. Then we can understand and address the problems that need to be solved.

CLINICAL VIGNETTE: THE OMEN

Steven was an adorable 4-year-old boy with a cute smile and bright red hair. His mother, Katherine, tall and slender with long, straight blonde hair, was in her early 30s, educated, and well versed in the principles of behavior modification. She explained in the first session that Steven, a normally sweet, gentle boy, had suddenly changed about 9 months earlier and had become aggressive toward his 18-month-old brother. Steven would hit his little brother and poke at his eyes and had even pushed him down the basement stairs on one occasion. The vast array of appropriate interventions Katherine had tried had all failed. She'd used time-outs, behavior charts, and restraint, and had talked to Steven about his feelings of anger. She described how Steven would suddenly get a crazed look in his eyes and seem possessed or act as if he had become another person.

What could cause such a transformation in a preschooler who ordinarily talks about his feelings and cuddles small animals? My first assumption was a routine one based on many cases that fit a common pattern. Katherine had divorced her husband 9 months previously as the result of his drinking. She stated clearly that, with the exception of his drinking, he had been a good husband and continued to be a good father. After the divorce Katherine had returned to school for a master's degree while continuing to work full-time as a speech therapist. Steven had been abruptly placed in day care for the first time in his life, and Katherine and her two boys had moved back into the home of her parents for both financial and moral support.

Because a therapist needs a working hypothesis, I explored all the important relationships involved, hoping to figure out what was causing Steven's violence. Katherine clearly stated that neither her ex-husband, mother, nor father presented any problems. She just had a wonderful boy who had become a monster. My first reaction was to presume that something was happening between Katherine and her ex-husband that was causing Steven to mediate their relationship in some way. Meanwhile, some relief from the immediate symptoms seemed in order. Katherine was clearly a gentle soul to whom violence was abhorrent. The more she tried to stop Steven from being aggressive, the more aggressive he became. This same dynamic was played out in a therapy session: When Steven began jumping on his chair, his mother spoke sweetly to him about not doing this; Steven did it even more. The more benevolent Katherine was, the more aggressive and disagreeable Steven became. Eventually, Steven hit his mother.

I decided to prescribe the metaphorical representation of the symptom (Madanes, 1981). Prescribing violence against others is unwise, so I asked Katherine to direct Steven to do to a stuffed animal what he did to his brother. (In this case a stuffed Garfield doll was handy, which seemed like an appropriate character to abuse.) I asked Katherine to insist that Steven kick, poke, beat, and push Garfield at least as cruelly as he hurt his brother. Both mother and child became noticeably anxious. They wound up talking about other things, and Katherine pursued a discussion of why they were in therapy. My directive to her to encourage Steven to attack the stuffed Garfield doll set up a new script in which Katherine would be insisting on violence in a safe context and Steven would be hesitant to comply. I directed them to do this exercise three times a day.

Accepting negative impulses and inclinations turned out to be quite difficult for Katherine. Her avoidance of overt anger reinforced my hypothesis that Steven was metaphorically telling us about his mother's anger at his father and offering her a proving ground on which to resolve that anger by curing Steven. When Steven and his mother returned 2 weeks later for their second session, little had changed. Katherine had spent a large portion of the allotted time directing Steven to kiss and make nice to Garfield after only brief moments of punching and kicking it. I then assigned a more structured form of the exercise for the next 2 weeks, and the change brought about a startling reaction. I told Katherine to have Steven spend 10 minutes abusing the doll after which he could make nice to it for 1 minute. Within a week there was a major crisis: Steven had begun swinging his fists at his grandfather when the man refused to give him more candy. When his grandfather tried to hold him and calm him down, Steven began kicking and spitting as well. Steven was so relentless in his attack that his grandfather had to pick him up and carry him into a room where he could leave the child alone and close the door.

After these attacks Katherine began discussing concerns she was having about the way her father was handling the boys and interfering with her parenting. Neither her mother nor father had lived with a small child for many years, and they became upset and corrected their grand-sons for harmless incivilities like leaving fingerprints on the glass coffee table. Katherine was genuinely upset about many of her parents' comments, but she couldn't allow herself to feel angry at her parents, who were putting their own lives on hold to help their only daughter after a divorce.

Once Katherine connected Steven's anger to her problem with her parents, the solution was simple. We scheduled a session when her parents could join us to negotiate boundaries and responsibilities for a grown daughter who was also a mother living in her parents' house. This session never took place. Katherine spontaneously discussed her needs with her parents, who were open and receptive to her requests. Following these discussions, Steven stopped his aggression toward his little brother. Katherine and Steven came for only a few more sessions—five in all. She wrote me a letter a year later saying that Steven and his brother were now sharing a room and that there had been no further violence beyond what she would consider normal for young siblings.

Steven's situation punctuates the urgency of the questions raised earlier in this chapter about young children. Are we looking at the metaphors and messages behind the symptoms in children, or are we searching for pathology? To a therapist focused on pathology, Steven was a terribly disturbed child who had demonstrated himself to be a serious danger to his brother by never missing an opportunity to hurt or injure a defenseless toddler. To a therapist interested in reading his symptom metaphorically, he was a child who was looking for a way for his (and his mother's) unacceptable anger to be recognized, channeled, and resolved. Steven's anger was stabilizing Katherine's relationship with her father rather than her ex-husband, and was the vehicle for understanding what was troubling his family and for getting those problems resolved. Perhaps children should be listened to more closely—on more than one level. By his actions, Steven was a demon, but the meaning behind those actions told us that he was a loyal son.

FRIGHTENING DIAGNOSES COMMONLY USED TO DESCRIBE CHILDREN

Character Disorder

Character disorder (i.e., explosive personality, narcissistic personality, or antisocial personality [sociopath]) describes people who have such a rigid view of the world that they respond with an inflexible defensive pattern that is believed to be unbreakable. People with explosive personality disorder have uncontrolled bouts of rage with no apparent explanation for the vehemence of their outbursts. They reportedly see nothing wrong with such outbursts of temper and always feel justified in their anger. If we insist on using this adult diagnosis to describe children, I feel certain this is the problem with my 3-year-old son. Although his fits look a lot like temper tantrums, I suspect the diagnosis of explosive personality disorder would fit also—though using this diagnosis is a lot like using a bazooka to kill a fly. I've treated many children with explosive tempers, and I must admit that some of their outbursts were awesome. Most such children improve in response to the time-honored wisdom of ignoring them, but using the diagnosis of explosive personality disorder is a first step toward the use of antidepressant or antipsychotic medication on small children.

Narcissistic personality disorder describes people who are so caught up in their own thoughts and feelings that they have no sense of what others may feel. This description fits my understanding of almost every child I've ever met under the age of 10. The conscience of a child seems to mature slowly, and helping their child develop sensitivity to others is an uphill struggle for most of the parents I know.

Antisocial personality disorder describes the more serious situation where a person fails to develop a conscience altogether. This person doesn't know right from wrong and will become a criminal. Again, values and morals are what we're socializing our children to develop over time. I wasn't aware that children are supposed to have succeeded at knowing right from wrong by 6 or 7 years of age. Many parents bring children to therapy for lying or stealing and for—what's even more alarming to them—showing no remorse at all. When looked at closely, the parents of such children are usually moralizing and lecturing at their kids constantly. Under these circumstances children learn rapidly that there's no need for them to think through what's right or wrong—since they'll be told again at any moment, anyway.

The problem with diagnosing a child or young adolescent with a character disorder is that such a diagnosis presumes that a child's personality is sufficiently formed to be accurately understood and described. I've found that children's personalities change at such a high rate that they're quite malleable. Childhood is a period of rapid growth and change. We should accept it as such, rather than believe we can take a clinical look at a moment in a child's life and know who he or she is and what he or she will become.

Bipolar Disorder or Manic–Depressive Illness

Manic depression is a diagnosis that describes an adult whose moods swing between profound depression and a stage of high energy and grandiosity. Most experts in the medical field believe that this condition is caused by a shortage of lithium in the brain and often describe manic depression as a genetically inherited disease. The use of lithium carbonate is usually the treatment of choice, but the condition is typically considered lifelong and incurable, with medication being required for the rest of the patient's life.

Over the last few years there has been a move in psychiatry to apply the diagnosis of bipolar disorder to young children and adolescents. Few of these children have identifiable drawn-out cyclical mood swings, and most are active and imaginative. The treatment of choice for children who carry this label is lithium carbonate and long-term talk therapy. It should be noted that lithium carbonate is sufficiently toxic that blood levels must be monitored regularly to ensure safety. It's unclear what long-term effects this drug has on developing minds and bodies. It's also unclear how children or parents are affected by being told that this incurable disease is probably inherited. I have yet to see conclusive evidence that a shortage of lithium causes bipolar symptoms or that the condition is inherited.

Schizophrenia

Although it is less common, there's a growing tendency to believe that children can become psychotic. Considering the vivid imagination of young children, it's difficult to differentiate between a hallucination and an invisible friend or monster under the bed. The greatest danger of a diagnosis of schizophrenia in a child is the use of psychotropic medications and the accompanying risk of neurological damage from them. Any professional applying such a diagnosis to a child should be viewed with a great deal of suspicion, and a second opinion should be sought.

Attention Deficit Disorder

In attempting to diagnose attention deficit disorder (ADD), we once again come up against the task of distinguishing between creativity and pathology. Literature is available on ADD that ranges from classifying it as a neurological disease to viewing it as a personal learning style that our society has trouble dealing with in a traditional classroom. The use of Ritalin (methylphenidate hydrochloride), a stimulant medication, is the number one method for dealing with children who have been diagnosed with ADD. Of interest is the fact that more boys than girls are being given a diagnosis of ADD. I wonder if this says something about the relative difficulty of socializing the aggressive tendencies in males and of compelling boys to fit into the regimentation of traditional school settings.

Even when ADD is the diagnosis, medication is used all too quickly for a disorder for which brief therapies are available that are effective in helping many of these children and their families. In addition, changes in the school setting often result in dramatic improvement in these children's functioning.

CONCLUSION

It's possible to describe a child's problems and intervene to ameliorate the symptoms without attaching a label to the child. A poster I once saw said LABEL JARS, NOT CHILDREN. (The good news is that in ADD, children finally have a disorder of their own, a diagnosis that was applied to them first and that is now being applied to adults, rather than the other way around.)

Although many childhood diagnoses within the American Psychiatric Association's *Diagnostic and Statistical Manual of Mental Disorders* are used daily, many childhood diagnoses are descriptive rather than indicative of pathology. When children with conduct disorder learn to conduct themselves properly, the description is no longer considered valid for them. Children with separation anxiety will be relieved of the anxiety when they adjust to the separation. These diagnoses simply aren't as stigmatizing or as lasting as the ones mentioned earlier, though calling any condition a "disorder" is still a harmful label.

The message to be passed on to parents is that they have every right to be suspicious of professionals who try to scare them into believing what doesn't make sense to them as parents and that they should question clinical conclusions that don't fit with their understanding of their own children. Professionals must be prepared to look at diagnostic formulas with suspicion; then, with fresh eyes, they must help parents look at their children as whole human beings who have the power, with the help of those who love them, to overcome adversity.

Parents' ability to stand firm in the face of professional opinion may at times be sorely challenged. Among the most stressful situations a parent can face is divorce. Other than death, there are few crises that can so totally disrupt a family's life, leading to parental weakness and uncertainty and to a variety of serious symptoms in family members. In the next chapter we will consider in detail the impact of divorce on adolescent aggression.

FOUR

When Divorce Conflict Causes Adolescent Aggression

Guilt, Loneliness, and Parents at War

AFTER THE DIVORCE: THE ROLES

A significant number of abusive young people come from families where there has been a divorce. Every therapist is familiar with the divorced mother whose child becomes her primary companion. A common image is a mother with a daughter who is her confidant and a son who is her nemesis; the son appears to replace a verbally abusive father, and the daughter continues an ongoing gender coalition with her mother. The nemesis is often an abusive teenager who gains additional power in the aftermath of a painful divorce. The confidant becomes powerful when a custodial parent who's upset by a painful divorce isn't getting proper adult emotional support and turns to a son or daughter for that support.

Although troubled family interactions after divorce aren't determined solely by gender, a pattern in which the child plays the role the same-sex parent played is most common. By filling the role of the missing parent, the child keeps the family locked in a struggle that makes it unnecessary to accept the finality of the divorce. As long as the parent's reaction to the child is similar to the reaction formerly reserved for the spouse, the child feels comfortable; that is, the child, reassured that the parents are still emotionally attached to each other, can keep an internal image of the continuation of the nuclear family he or she is having trouble giving up.

A Fictional Vignette: Role Confusion

What type of divorce is the breeding ground for the development of an aggressive adolescent or young adult? One of the most common accompaniments of a painful divorce is the litany of blame. The battle establishing blame begins long before the divorce is final and often intensifies as a child becomes progressively more allied with one parent in blaming the other. Such a situation is graphically portrayed in the novel *Ordinary People*, (Guest, 1976). The following excerpt from that novel (pp. 109–112) walks the reader through a three-way conflict that's so vivid it could easily be a true situation. The parents have just discovered that their son had been skipping swim practice and had then quit the team altogether weeks earlier. Because Conrad has developed psychiatric symptoms, his parents are confused about how tough to be. Through his depression Conrad is attacking his mother, Beth. This is a classic case of a child who abuses his parents by developing psychiatric symptoms. The excerpt begins with Conrad's father, Cal, challenging him about where he was when he wasn't at swim practice.

"Where have you been every night?" he asks.

"Nowhere," Conrad says. "Around. The library, mostly."

"I don't get it," he says flatly. "Why didn't you tell us?"

"I was going to. I've been meaning to—"

"I'm sure you would have told us before the first meet," Beth says. "When is it, next Thursday?"

"I'm sure I would have told you," Conrad says, "if I thought you gave a damn!"

And the wellspring of anger erupts, engulfing them all.

"What the hell does that mean?" Cal demands.

"Never mind," she says. "It's meant for me. Isn't it? I wish I knew, Conrad, why it is still so important for you to try to hurt me!"

"Hurt you? Me hurt you! Listen, you're the one who's trying to hurt me!"

"And how did I do that? By making you look like a fool in front of a roomful of people? Did you have to sit there, getting those looks? Poor Mrs. Jarrett, oh the poor woman, she has no idea what her son is up to, he lies and lies and she believes every word of it—"

"I didn't lie—"

"You did! You lied every night that you came into this house at six-thirty. What do you mean, you didn't lie?" She presses her hands tight to her head. "I can't stand this, I really can't! If it's starting all over again, the lying and the disappearing for hours, the covering up—I won't stand it!"

"Don't then!" he snarls. "Go to Europe, why don't you? Go to hell!"

"Con—"

But he backs away from Cal's hand. "Listen, don't give me that, the only reason you care, the only reason you give a *fuck* about it is because someone else knew about it first! You never wanted to know anything I was doing, or anything I *wasn't* doing; you just wanted me to leave you alone! Well, I left you alone, didn't I? I could have told you lots of things! Like, up at the hospital there were rats! Big ones, up on three, with the hopeless nuts! But that's okay; see, I was down on two, with the heads and the unsuccessfuls—"

Until this point in the conversation Conrad was alluding to a conflict between his parents over his mother's being away during his hospitalization. He had good reason to be angry at both parents for not protecting him from abuse in a psychiatric hospital, yet he was directing his rage only toward his mother. A reader can regard this excerpt from the book as an expression of Conrad's feelings toward his mother— which is the way his parents understood it—or as a straightforward account of parents learning their son had lied to them. As the conversation continues it becomes harder for the reader to figure out whether the conflict is between Conrad's parents or just about him. Is this a discussion of a child's dishonesty or a glimpse of a long-standing conflict in a marriage? Cal's failure to defend his wife puts him in a coalition with his son against her. As the conversation continues, Conrad gets himself more and more deeply embedded between his parents as he focuses his accusations on his mother and says things to her that his father wishes he could say.

"Con, shut up, stop it—"
"Damn it!" he says. "Tell *her* to stop it! You never tell her a *goddamn thing!* Listen, I know why she never came out there, not once! *I know!* Hell, she was going to goddamn *Spain* and goddamn *Portugal*, why should she care if I was hung up by the *goddamn balls* out there—"
"Christ! That's enough!"
He takes a swift, sobbing breath, fixing them both with a look of utter fury. And then he is gone, his feet pounding up the stairs. Moments later, the shattering slam of his bedroom door.
Beth has her back to Cal, her hands clutching at her head. "I won't, I won't!"
He goes to her; puts his arms around her. Her body is stiff. She is trembling, but she does not relax against him.
"What happened?" he asks. "What the hell happened?"
"I don't know!"
"Somebody'd better go up there."
"Go!" she says. "Go ahead, that's the pattern, isn't it? Let him walk all over us, then go up there and apologize to him!"
"I'm not going to apologize."

"Yes you are! You always do! You've been apologizing to him ever since he came home!"

"Ah, Beth, crissake, lay off, will you? I feel like I've been at a goddamn tennis match tonight! Back and forth, back and forth—"

"Don't talk to me like that!" She twists violently away from him. "Don't talk to me like he talks to you!"

"Let's go upstairs," he says.

"No. You go. He wants you. He wants somebody who's going to accept everything he does. Without question, without criticism . . . "

"And you think that's what I do?"

"I know it is!"

"I think," he says cautiously, "that there might have been a better way to handle this."

"Oh, I'm sure of it." Her voice is bitter. "For openers, he could have come to us and told us the truth."

"No, I meant tonight."

"I know what you meant! You see? Everything he does is all right! Perfectly understandable! And everything I do is—is mixed up, and wrong, and could have been handled a better way!"

"That's not true! That's not what I'm trying to say!"

His nerves are raw. His eyes feel as if they have sunk back into his head, pulling the flesh down. "Beth. Please. Let's just go upstairs!"

"No! I will not be pushed!" she says. She moves away from him to stand before the window, looking out. Calmly she says, "I will not be *manipulated*."

Beth acts as if she and Conrad were rivals trying to get Cal's approval. This lack of definition of appropriate roles is typical of struggles in which a marital conflict centers around a symptomatic child. In this case the father is in the role of mediator between his wife and his son—again, as if mother and son were equals. The story ends with Beth moving out of the house as Conrad's psychiatric symptoms improve. If Beth and Cal go on to divorce, the situation has the potential for their son's developing serious problems with aggression in the future. Battle lines were drawn between parents who would have to deal with each other to help their children for years to come despite their anger.

AFTER THE DIVORCE: THE FEELINGS

No matter how convinced parents are that they're doing the right thing by divorcing, there's always a small voice in their head accusing them of breaking up their family, either by driving their partner away or by leaving the marriage. These voices of self-doubt and guilt may be intensified by children who deliver the same powerful accusations when they're un-happy with how their parents are handling things. It's particularly powerful for a child to point out that the other parent would never handle things so poorly and that if it weren't for this parent's part in causing the divorce, there would be no problems at all. In the early months and years of readjustment following a divorce, parents are particularly vulnerable to such attacks. Their guilt may rise rapidly as their self-doubt increases in response to attacks by their children, ex-spouse, or a combination of the two.

As parents become more doubtful, adolescents become more power-ful. Parents become more and more focused on their inner pain and their anger at children who keep throwing salt on the wounds. Children of divorced parents learn that they get more freedom and less parental control when they incapacitate their parents with guilt-provoking words. Divorced people who were abused by their spouse during the marriage or who were abused during childhood may become even more incapacitated by their child's threats of violence.

Typically, children whose parents divorce have watched them sys-tematically try to destroy each other during the divorce process. As the custodial parent flounders in pain after the divorce, some children become a confidant in order to make the parent's daily life more bearable or try to entertain the parent by becoming a companion. They may help in practical ways, for example, by taking care of younger children. They may even challenge the parent to stop being self-pitying.

Such children anxiously watch as a beloved parent exudes guilt, shame, sadness, and loneliness. These feelings are so loud that the young person feels compelled to make vigorous efforts to save the parent from turning inward and shutting out the world. When these efforts to break through the parent's shell fail to help, adolescents begin to accept the parent's withdrawal and their helplessness to reverse it, but they gain power and autonomy in the process; after all, it's hard to supervise an adolescent from inside a shell. Teenagers who fail to help depressed parents after a divorce may tell their parents and therapists that they can now do whatever they want and that there's nothing their parents can do to stop them. If parents threaten punishment, adolescents simply refuse the punishment. If parents threaten to physically stop them from leaving the house without permission, teenagers in turn threaten to report the parents to the authorities for abuse. Parents whose level of self-confidence is at an all-time low believe what their sons and daughters are saying and can be controlled by words alone.

Parents at this stage of divorce often stop seeing anyone outside the family, which only makes the situation worse. Their own parents and friends may withdraw to avoid becoming entangled in the divorce strug-gle, or they may become critical or patronizing—others often believe that if they were in the same situation, they would handle it better. When divorced parents finally try to have a relationship with someone of the opposite sex, their children may make it so difficult for them, by mistreating their dates, that the parents eventually give up trying to develop relationships. One could contend that because it's been so stressful for these children to see a parent in such terrible pain, they feel they must assume a protective role by standing between the parent and anyone who might cause further pain. Like a bird that won't come out of its cage even though the door is left open, some parents eventually accept their helplessness to escape these daily struggles and become convinced that they lack the necessary energy to do anything but contend with their children.

Some depressed parents in postdivorce struggles may explain their lethargy as the result of having to deal with an overprotective or even an abusive teenager, just as they may have attributed all of their past difficulties to the errant spouse's transgressions. Although it's true that some children do make it difficult for a divorced parent to resume a social life, the loneliness of living without a partner and the insecurity that accompanies attempts to reenter the dating scene are pretty discouraging under the best of conditions.

Feelings of guilt and remorse after divorce are heavily rooted in American culture. The American legal system is finally giving up its prerogative to tell couples whether they may or may not be granted a divorce. Despite this progress the courts still treat divorce in an adversarial manner, implying that divorce is a sign of moral weakness on the part of one of the spouses. Courts still demonstrate whose "fault" the divorce is by making it their job to determine who the best parent is. At times, divorce seems more like a criminal rather than a civil matter because punishment is meted out. The confusion gets worse when the court assumes so much control over parents' rights in a contentious divorce that its permission must be obtained for many major decisions. The court becomes a permanent member of the family after divorce. Thus, parents not only may feel uncertain about their ability to competently handle their children but may not even have the legal right to try.

Meanwhile, the more helpless a parent becomes in response to an unsupportive system, the more ammunition an ex-spouse has for demonstrating that that person is an unfit parent. This struggle of evidence and defense usually results in noncustodial parents feeling that they must prove their worth. To this end they petition the court every couple of years to publicly demonstrate that the previous rulings are wrong and that their ex-spouse is really the bad parent. Unfortunately, the adversarial nature of this struggle set up by the courts perpetuates aggression in children by modeling the need for winners and losers. As the children respond to the model, custodial parents look even worse because they have children who are out of control.

In summary, parents embedded in postdivorce misery become paralyzed on a variety of levels. Their children may become emotionally abusive; they feel guilty for having deprived their children of an intact family; and they are punished by an adversarial court system whose purpose is to assign blame, which only increases the guilt and shame of those who already doubt themselves. Their sense of guilt, which may be exacerbated by other family members, is made worse by their growing loneliness. Moreover, the loneliness drags on because prospective mates stop calling when they realize what a mess they'd be getting themselves into by becoming involved with someone who has a troubled child and an angry ex-spouse.

CLINICAL VIGNETTE: PAIN IN THE POSTDIVORCE STRUGGLE

Alexis was a 32-year-old woman whose divorce was complete except for the court's findings in the child custody dispute. Her son, Kevin, was 8 and her daughter, Lydia, was 6 at the time of the divorce. Her ex-husband was granted temporary custody of the children, and she was allowed visitation every other weekend and one evening a week. Her ex-husband was financially very well off while she was going to be living on a secretary's income with no child support. In fact, Alexis would be paying child support to her husband. This was a problem for her because, although she could draw money from the divorce settlement for living expenses, she wanted to save as much as possible to pay for college for the children.

Alexis found it humiliating being a noncustodial mother and became depressed and angry. People accused her of giving up her children when, in fact, she'd fought hard for them and lost. She began having arguments with Kevin. These arguments were the main point her ex-husband used in court to justify limiting her involvement with their son. Kevin became more angry and verbally abusive when he was with Alexis and repeated things he'd heard his father say to criticize her. Meanwhile, Lydia and Alexis got along well and became very close. Alexis's obvious pleasure and pride in Lydia only increased Kevin's anger at his mother.

Kevin's father decided to put him in individual therapy to help with his emotional problems. Alexis was never seen by that therapist. This is a formula for disaster. When serious conflict in a family pushes people into individual therapies, the people involved become more and more polarized and the anger gets worse. Since Kevin's father had full legal custody of him, Alexis wasn't consulted on the choice of therapist. Yet it seems that the subject of that therapy was primarily Kevin's anger at his mother. As his therapy continued, the boy criticized his mother more frequently and even pushed her on two occasions.

When Alexis arranged for a rehearing of the custody decision, Kevin's therapist testified that the boy shouldn't see his mother because the relationship was too destructive. In his testimony the therapist repeated statements Kevin had made during sessions about wanting his mother dead, statements that had clearly been led by the interviewer. Fortunately, the judge made a sensible decision to gradually rebuild Alexis' relationship with Kevin. However, doing so continued to be difficult. Alexis spent more time with Lydia than with Kevin because her son was difficult to deal with and his father did what he could to interfere with the visitation. As Alexis's guilt and shame about being a "bad mother" grew, she became more depressed and began having trouble exercising enough self-control to keep from taking her anger at her ex-husband out on Kevin. Meanwhile, Kevin continued to argue with her in a way that resembled what he had seen of his father's behavior toward his mother during the divorce.

It took Alexis years to learn to see Kevin as a child again rather than as a younger version of her abusive ex-spouse. On the other hand, when Lydia became an adolescent and began asserting herself, Alexis was able to see her as a typical child who wanted her way.

THE REMARRIED PARENT WITH AN AGGRESSIVE TEENAGER

When a divorced parent remarries, after managing to find and nurture a relationship with someone who has the perseverance to stick with an obviously difficult situation, new problems arise. The relationship between a teenager and a new stepparent usually takes one of two forms.

The Head-to-Head Struggle

Some adolescents hate the new stepparent and engage in a power struggle that begins immediately after the wedding. The son or daughter relentlessly continues a verbal and emotional assault until the stepparent is doing and saying things the biological parent doesn't approve of. The parent, who has already practiced feeling guilty about the child's fate for many months, now feels even worse. As the stepparent becomes angrier and more negative, the parent may come to believe that the child's life has been ruined by the decision to remarry.

It must be noted that in many remarriage situations the new step-parent may have started out handling things reasonably well only to have his or her conduct and resolve slowly deteriorate under the onslaught mounted by the abusive stepchild. The stepparent may have respected the biological parent's moral right to be in charge of the child and may have intervened only after witnessing so much abuse of others that it was impossible to continue ignoring it.

Once a stepparent begins usurping the authority of the biological parent, the teenager explodes and the biological parent withdraws into feelings of guilt and inadequacy. There may also be a competitive non-custodial parent who secretly supports the child's assault on the new intruder into the family system.

The Helpful Stepparent

A second possible situation results when the stepparent marries the helpless parent of an aggressive child or adolescent in order to rescue both parent and child. A stepfather may presume that all the young person needs is the strong hand that only a man can provide. The strategy of a stepfather who sees himself as a knight in shining armor usually deterio-rates rapidly when the power tactics of the teenager incapacitate him as effectively as they did the mother. The stepfather may then turn on his new wife for being such a lousy parent, which further humiliates her and reduces the chances that she'll ever take charge. The stepdad, however well intentioned, is now stuck in the knight in shining armor scenario. He's tried being the benevolent friend and also the firm authority figure to no avail. Now that the dragon is winning, the knight blames the maiden he's trying to rescue because she shouldn't have gone out of the castle in the first place. Again, the mother's guilt becomes even greater as her new husband, who she thought was on her side, attacks her for her lack of strength.

A new stepmother is more likely to feel her stepchildren need understanding rather than the rigid punitive posture their biological father has assumed. She tries to be the loving mother to children damaged by divorce and is rapidly neutralized by the children's power tactics. She is devastated by the fact that the children either are unresponsive or laugh in her face, and she may turn on her husband, blaming him for getting her into this mess. The new stepmother often becomes the primary parent, and the father may leave the job to her once it becomes clear that she's willing to do it. The stepmother then becomes angry at both father and children. The father's guilt over taking his children away from their mother then skyrockets because he feels he has now failed to provide them with a stepmother who could have neutralized the effects of the divorce (thereby assuaging his own guilt) by developing a loving relationship with them.

The Wicked Stepmother

Michael and Jane, his second wife, spoke with me after Michael's 17-year-old daughter, Maria, moved out of the house to live with a friend's family, leaving her 6-year-old sister without a sibling at home. Michael described a constant struggle between stepdaughter and stepmother because of Maria's insolence and Jane's lack of understanding and acceptance of the girl's point of view. Because Michael had a history of exploding when dealing with Maria, Jane had assumed the pivotal task of trying to correct Maria's misbehaviors. When Jane turned to Michael for help, he was likely to either overreact or do little, and there was no way to predict which response would occur.

Michael and Jane had agreed that Maria would soon be going to live with her biological mother for the summer. The question they raised in therapy was where Maria would live in the fall. Michael wanted to either have her live on her own without bad feelings between them, or work out a way to integrate her into the family. Jane, for her part, had thrown up her hands in frustration and had told Michael to handle the situation. Michael continued to live in fear of retribution from both his daughter and his new wife. He felt that if he took any decisive action, one of them would be unhappy with whatever he did.

The situation presented by Michael, Jane, and Maria is a classic example of a loving stepmother—who in this case happened to be a social worker—intent on helping an apparently helpless father raise his daughter. Michael became progressively less effective with Maria as Jane took over, and Jane herself became progressively more intolerant of the teenager as her attempts to help her were thwarted by Maria and not appreciated by Michael. Maria had increased her misbehavior to the point where this unhealthy triangle could no longer continue. Her behavior forced her father and stepmother to come together and begin planning rather than merely reacting.

Michael, Jane, and Maria entered the first therapy session resigned to their conclusion that Maria would never be able to live with her father and stepmother again. They assumed that Maria would have to either move into her own apartment or continue living with a friend. The emotions underlying this family drama were complicated by the fact that

Maria's biological mother had never forgiven her for moving in with her father instead of with her. Maria's mother said things designed to make the teenager feel guilty, a feeling that hindered her ability to be patient and adjust to her father's new marriage.

When I asked each family member to be frank in their discussion about living arrangements for Maria in the fall, Maria admitted that she preferred to live with her dad and stepmother. Jane replied that she wanted to feel like a successful stepmother. Michael said he was mortified by the idea of Maria moving out. Once each party admitted to wanting the family back together, the injured feelings each had developed began settling down. I was able to help parents and child negotiate a set of guidelines that were more age appropriate than some of the expectations Michael had of Maria. The family allowed me to direct them because I stood firm against each family member's threats of emotional explosion and didn't avoid important points. I convinced each member to say and do small positive things that could help reduce the conflict. I pushed parents and young adult alike to say the positive things about each other that I knew they felt but that their rigid positions in the struggle hadn't allowed them to say.

Jane turned out to be Maria's advocate, encouraging Michael to be less worried and overcontrolling; she was able to advise him without taking over the primary parenting role for herself. Michael was able to risk trusting Maria more, and Maria worked with her father and step-mother to honor agreements she'd made. Maria even went out of her way to be helpful around the house and babysit for her 6-year-old sister. The babysitting was a major concession because Jane had sworn in the first session that she'd never trust Maria to tend her sister again because she'd been irresponsible in the past.

The therapy succeeded because a "choreographer"—the therapist— was hired to organize who would play what roles in a stepfamily situation. Michael regained his position as father and took responsibility for dealing with his daughter. Jane assumed the role of learned consultant who offered him invaluable knowledge about dealing with a teenage girl. Maria learned how to relate to a stepmother by learning that a stepmother needn't act like a biological parent. All three said they never expected to see the loving side of the others, which was now so clearly visible to them.

The therapy took seven sessions. In addition to the family reorgani-zation, intervention included helping Michael deal appropriately with his ex-wife. In the past he'd seen Maria's problems with her mother as an issue only between the two of them and not his concern, an approach that had left Maria alone to handle problems her parents wanted to avoid talking about. Finally, Maria exploded and her parents were forced to begin dealing with each other. By the end of therapy, Maria, whose unresolved problems were typical of the children of postdivorce families, no longer had to cause crises to draw attention to her needs.

With postdivorce conflict more the rule than the exception, parents must ask themselves what they can do to prevent their children from becoming troubled in the wake of a bitter divorce. Let us now look closely at how our culture views divorce and consider what can be done to change the way divorce is handled.

PREVENTING POSTDIVORCE AGGRESSION THROUGH THERAPY

The more I deal with divorce, the more strongly I feel that it isn't taken seriously enough. When people get married, there's a big celebration with uplifting religious and cultural rituals to help with the adjustment. When they divorce, they're just not married anymore; most of the rituals associated with divorce aren't exactly uplifting or supportive. Marriage comes with inflated expectations smacking of fairy-tale endings; it's seen as a positive, wonderful event. Divorce, on the other hand, is seen as a failure. Both partners feel guilty and ashamed and may not get nearly the love and support from family and friends that they were given when they were married and that they need even more now. Could this be part of the reason so many people come to therapy legally divorced but still emotionally married? Couples may be acting married 10 years after their divorce is final. In fact, a large percentage of problems with aggressive teenagers originate in a divorce. It follows, then, that if we can help people have healthier divorces, we can reduce the rate of teenage aggression.

Understanding the dilemma of divorce holds the key to treating (1) the divorced parent who must now raise an angry, abusive child single-handedly, and (2) the remarried couple who must deal with the anger of a child who has lost one parent to divorce and must learn to live with a stepparent. An understanding of divorce not only gives therapists clues to helping families who remain in distress after the divorce but also enables them to make the process of divorce a more tolerable and cooperative experience for their clients, thereby reducing the intensity of the problems that may show up later in treatment.

Carl Whitaker (1989) referred to families as organisms. A family's covert rules and cybernetic interactions connect its members in ways we can't see or easily understand. Whitaker once said that he knows this connection exists because his children's faces are the only ones he can look into and see both himself and his wife. If the family is an organism, then it would feel like an amputation for a portion of it to be suddenly removed. An understanding of the organic nature of attachment in families makes it difficult to view a marriage as something that just dies, with one or both spouses walking away from it with a relieved sigh. This organic view also explains why some people in miserable marriages don't want to let go. Maybe they know something.

In an organism each part works cooperatively and in the best interest of the whole organism. Family members, too, work together in a unified way to fight whatever threatens the family's stability, whatever seems like an infection or disease in the marriage. The fact that what they're doing isn't working doesn't mean that their intentions are subversive. So why do unhappily married people continue hurting each other instead of retreating happily?

Is it possible that troubled spouses are trying to help each other right to the very end of the marriage—and sometimes beyond? Family members' attempts to continue helping loved ones demonstrate the persistence of the human spirit. Even in the face of defeat, couples have a hard time giving up. Perhaps unhappy couples in the process of divorcing are still trying to solve the same problems they wanted to solve to save their marriage. This continuing need to solve past marital problems could explain why the spouse of an alcoholic has trouble leaving as long as the alcoholic is still killing him- or herself with alcohol. In many cases one or both spouses have undertaken a mission to help the other, for example, by pulling the other out of a severe depression or by bringing a workaholic back into the family. Evidence that this mission is accomplished is a change in the errant mate's behavior in the direction the other desires.

In a divorce situation, neither person's role or mission has changed except that the energy formerly devoted to changing the other to save the marriage is directed to the task of getting a divorce. Consider, for example, a case in which one spouse has repeatedly tried to pull the other out of a depression by launching a verbal attack specifically for the purpose of activating the other's anger. This verbal aggression then evolves into physical abuse (this is by no means intended as an explanation for all physical abuse)—a development that does nothing, of course, to improve the marriage or help the spouse's depression. The situation deteriorates further, and the couple decide to divorce. The "helpful" spouse, who hoped the decision to divorce would improve matters, now has to understand why the other is being so difficult in the divorce process. The most reasonable explanation is that the other is still depressed. This realization reactivates the "helpful" spouse's need to attempt to intervene in that depression. If this pattern in the divorce process isn't interrupted, after the divorce the depressed parent may find that the child has learned the same pattern of intrusive helpfulness exhibited by the ex-spouse—a behavior that can escalate into adolescent abusiveness. If the adolescent becomes abusive, the "helpful" parent may applaud the abusive behavior and may blame the violence on the depressed ex-spouse. This abusive cycle between parent and child mimics the pattern the spouses had in the marriage. Despite the obvious futility of continuing an unsuccessful pattern of behavior, people rarely give up on a problem-solving technique in which they've invested time and effort. Before a child's behavior reaches the stage of parent abuse, the therapist must unravel the same pattern of behavior that existed in the marriage but with different players. In other words, the story is one of a troubled marriage that leads to a divorce and then evolves into a parent abuse case.

Clinical Vignette

How does a therapist find a useful solution when the struggle between a married couple continues into the divorce phase? I observed one such couple from behind the one-way mirror during a therapy session that included their teenage daughter. The therapist was an experienced social worker named Chris Protonotarios who was participating in an intensive live-supervision training program. In live supervision the therapist is observed by a supervisor through a one-way mirror to teach and assist. The supervisor can call into the session by phone to offer suggestions or observations.

Mr. and Mrs. Hunter came to this first session presenting their 18-year-old daughter, Gina, as their major concern. Gina, who lived with her mother, was slim and poised and spoke well. Her manner contrasted with that of her parents. Mrs. Hunter, thin with angular features, fidgeted nervously while her somewhat overweight husband leaned back in his chair in a corner of the room and looked sullen. Gina sat between her mother and father.

Mrs. Hunter described her daughter as being too dependent on her boyfriend and as disrespectful and emotionally abusive because of her tendency to argue with and browbeat her. Mrs. Hunter claimed that Gina took endlessly from her by using her emotional vulnerability as a woman facing divorce to get whatever she wanted. Gina told Chris that she was graduating from high school with a 3.8 grade point average and intended to go away to college in the fall.

Before the interview could focus more clearly on Gina, Mr. Hunter brought up the fact that he and his wife were in the process of getting a divorce. Before Chris could get more details, Mr. and Mrs. Hunter began arguing bitterly about their impending divorce. Their complaints about Gina disappeared for the moment. I could see that this was a parent abuse case waiting to happen. As the supervisor behind the one-way-mirror, I was concerned about how rapidly tempers were escalating. Gina tried to calm everyone by lecturing her mother and touching her father's shoulder to comfort him. I called into the room and suggested to Chris that he challenge both parents about how intensely involved with each other they seemed to be. I recommended that he discuss how they were ever going to let go of each other enough to get divorced with such emotional attachment going on.

Chris began, "You argue like people who still want to be involved . . . married, that is."

Mrs. Hunter leaned forward in tears and said, "No, not married. I don't want to be married. I've never been divorced. What do divorced people do? I don't know!"

Hoping to get some support for the idea that they were intimately attached, Chris turned to Gina, who was sitting between her parents, and asked, "Is this like the way they reacted to each other when they were together?"

"Yeah, they've always been like this," she answered.

Chris continued, "Sounds like people who want to stay married."

Mr. Hunter continued to sit in the corner with a tolerant look on his face as his wife continued in her dramatic tone of voice: "He just withholds. All he does is withhold. He withholds his presents. He withholds any information he has. He lies to me! He doesn't tell me the truth. He withholds all the things he says he's going to do. He says he's going to do them, but he never does them. He withholds! He withholds! I used to believe him. I don't believe him anymore."

As Mrs. Hunter continued, Gina patted her father's leg and muttered to her mother, "You don't have to let him."

I was beginning to think Mrs. Hunter was trapped by her own attempts to change her husband. The things she was accusing him of in the marriage were now making it difficult for her to get a divorce. Mr. Hunter was sitting without expression or response during her tirade, which confirmed to me her comments about his withholding nature.

Mrs. Hunter continued trying to get herself unstuck from what seemed like a helpless position: "What are divorced people supposed to do? Tell me and I'll try to act that way. How am I supposed to act to get out of this marriage? Because I don't want to be married to him. He hurts me! Every time I'm with him. It tears me up to be around him!"

Chris did a nice job of weaving what Mrs. Hunter was saying back into his clinical position by saying, "Gina said this is the way you both behaved toward each other while you were living together. You're mad at him now like you were then."

Mrs. Hunter confirmed the trap she was in by finishing with, "He won't do anything we have to do to get this resolved! He won't . . . oh shit . . . he controls everything." Then, in a calmer voice, she said, "I'll try to get divorced. How do you do this?"

Chris challenged the divorcing couple to act in a new way. The Hunters are an example of a pattern in which the husband withholds and the wife lambastes him for withholding, which increases his withholding, which increases her outrage and recriminations. Their marriage had operated this way for 20 years, and no apparent change had occurred as a result of the separation and impending divorce.

Who, then, was helping whom? Mr. Hunter had been deeply depressed; he had been hospitalized 6 months before this session after trying to hang himself. His suicide attempt followed a serious financial setback in his company. I wondered whether Mrs. Hunter's reactivity to her husband and her emotional struggles with him were keeping him from lapsing back into a suicidal depression. Mr. Hunter certainly had a depressed look about him.

My hunch that Mrs. Hunter was helping her husband was supported by the revelation that she made ongoing trips to his house to take him cough medicine when he was sick. I wondered whether Mrs. Hunter would have any purpose in life if she no longer felt compelled to focus all of her thoughts and actions on her husband. Needless to say, the situation was ripe for their daughter to become a martyred companion to her father or an emotional abuser in her relationship with her mother—or both.

I was pleased with having found an understanding of the problem that fit the facts of the case. Understanding alone wasn't enough to warrant calling the process therapy, though. The challenge now was to do something to improve the situation.

Chris acknowledged Gina's kindness in trying to help her parents but suggested that she remove herself from their struggle because it would soon be time for her to go away to college. "I appreciate the fact that you're trying to help your mother to understand, but it sounds like it hasn't worked," Chris began.

Gina answered, "I can't help her so I just leave her alone for a while and then she'll calm down."

Chris repeated, "So it hasn't worked." Then he asked, "How about letting me deal with these things for a while?" Gina nodded in response.

Chris and I consulted behind the mirror to decide on a strategy for breaking the impasse created by the destructive, repetitive emotional struggle that characterized the Hunters' marriage. Chris and I decided that he would challenge whether or not the couple was truly ready for a divorce.

When Chris returned to the treatment room, he made the following remarks to Mr. and Mrs. Hunter: "It's clear to me that the two of you still feel a lot of love for one another. If you were to begin to cooperate with each other on the terms of the divorce, you would begin to feel better and better about each other. As that happened, your love for each other would become amplified, which would make it impossible for the two of you to get divorced. Your renewed love will result in the two of you continuing to experience the pain you've described for many more years. For now, I think you should not work so hard to achieve cooperation because if you were to succeed, your problems with one another could become more fierce and bind you together even more painfully."

Mrs. Hunter wrung her hands saying there must be something they could do to achieve cooperation and complete the divorce. Mr. Hunter leaned forward for the first time and agreed that there must be a way to work out the divorce. Having gotten a positive response, Chris reluctantly agreed that if they insisted, they could attempt to agree on the resolution of one small controversial item in their divorce. Chris warned them that if their interaction became emotionally passionate during the next 2 weeks (the interval between the first and second therapy sessions), they must stop trying to agree, because their love for each other was again becoming overwhelming.

Many therapists respond to interventions like the one Chris used with a great deal of doubt. They claim that if they said this to couples they treat, those couples would laugh in their face. In fact, they don't laugh when the therapist's intervention fits the facts the couple have shared with the therapist. Mrs. Hunter really was bringing Mr. Hunter chicken soup, and he was trying to leave his life insurance policy to her after the divorce.

It's important to track the nonverbal messages that spouses transmit in response to such an intervention. From the very beginning of Chris's talk about their intense love, both Mr. and Mrs. Hunter were nodding affirmatively in response to each statement. They were nonverbally telling Chris to continue on his current course. If they'd argued with Chris, I would have directed him to point out how the discussion they were having about their attempts to divorce mimicked those throughout their marriage. He could also have repeated things they said during the session that were evidence of their continued attachment.

The following transcript demonstrates the state of the Hunters' relationship when they returned 2 weeks later for their next therapy session. The goal had been to interrupt the cycle of passionate attachment between them so that they could either proceed with their divorce or rediscover each other in a more positive way.

Both Mr. and Mrs. Hunter walked into the second session looking pleased. Both sat forward in their chairs, and the sense of impending doom that had filled the therapy room 2 weeks earlier was gone. Chris began by asking, "Where's Gina?"

Surprisingly, Mr. Hunter answered first, saying, "She decided that her presence wasn't needed, and we—"

Mrs. Hunter completed his sentence with, "We're working on our divorce, and she doesn't need to be involved with that because she's got enough problems—and when we get back to talking about that, that's fine—right now. Last week it was all us with her in the middle, and it seems that's where she's been for some time."

Mr. Hunter added, "She felt very uncomfortable."

The degree to which we'd removed Gina from the triangle with her parents was far beyond what we had hoped, so it seemed reasonable to push ahead and see if the couple had made any progress on negotiating their divorce.

Chris said, "Did you try to work out one of the issues in the divorce, as we discussed?"

Mrs. Hunter replied, "Yes, our taxes. And this is what we're working on today. We've worked on them, but we aren't getting ready to do them yet." Mrs. Hunter turned to her husband and made eye contact with him while asking him a question. He responded in what looked like a kindly fashion.

Maintaining his pose of having only reluctantly agreed to let them try solving a problem together, Chris asked the couple, "How do you know when to start working on this issue?"

Mrs. Hunter said, "Well, we've collected all the stuff and—"

Mr. Hunter completed her sentence, saying, "Now we just have to take it to an accountant."

Mrs. Hunter then turned to Mr. Hunter and said, "You better write yourself a note." Mr. Hunter reached into his pocket and took out a pen to make a note of the suggestion. Then Mrs. Hunter turned back to Chris, saying, "The ball is in his court now because he has some kind of stock."

Mr. Hunter explained, "It's a real estate partnership, and it makes the taxes a bit more confused because of the tax shelters. Not everybody knows how to handle it. I'm going to take it, but I haven't been up to doing almost anything for the past week and a half."

Surprisingly, Mrs. Hunter defended her husband by verifying his statement: "He's been home in bed. He hasn't been at work or anything."

Outcome and Discussion

Mr. and Mrs. Hunter had responded to the challenge put to them by their therapist. Not only had they stopped fighting, but Mrs. Hunter defended her husband when it came out that he hadn't done his part in completing a task. The fact that this couple was proceeding with their settlement negotiations rather than falling back into each other's arms suggests that a divorce was truly what they were seeking but they had been too emotionally entwined to proceed with it. Their therapist again chal-lenged the couple by wondering aloud how they'd succeeded in working together to address a divorce issue when he'd predicted that they wouldn't be able to take additional steps without their love for each other getting in the way. They both acted as if they didn't know how they'd done it.

We scheduled sessions for the Hunters every other week. Each session demonstrated further resolution of the issues needed to complete the divorce. The couple discussed and agreed on a range of financial issues. They examined Mr. Hunter's plan to assign his soon-to-be ex-wife as the beneficiary of his life insurance. Chris attempted to set a proper boundary by suggesting that Mr. Hunter leave his policy to Gina and name Mrs. Hunter to supervise its use. Together the couple worked out various practical issues related to the divorce, including how their debts would be divided, how Gina's college would be paid for, and where she would stay during breaks from college. As the Hunters successfully negotiated these issues, Chris indicated that he was being proven "wrong" in his initial assessment of them by gradually expressing less doubt about their love for each other interfering with their progress.

After the Hunters' sixth therapy session, the court date arrived and their divorce was finalized. All of the settlement issues were resolved to the satisfaction of both Mr. and Mrs. Hunter. The therapy ended at this point and was resumed 3 months later, when Mr. and Mrs. Hunter sought help agreeing to the terms of Gina's move away to college. Mrs. Hunter returned again after Gina left for college for assistance in adjusting to this new stage in her daughter's life and in getting on with her own life.

When used properly, the therapist's decision to approach change skeptically generates an interesting discussion. On one level the therapist's skepticism is a challenge. More importantly, the discussion is an opportu-nity for clients to consider how hard the change process is and how tempting it is to stop expending the energy needed to continue changing.

PREVENTING POSTDIVORCE AGGRESSION THROUGH SOCIAL RITUAL

In addition to therapeutic interventions designed to disrupt the rigid pattern of interaction a couple is engaged in, a great deal can be accom-plished by utilizing the power of ritual to help people let go of their painful pasts. Our culture offers certain rituals to help couples extricate themselves from each other. Although the most popular rituals for divorce are at times effective, they can also be quite bloody.

The most well known rituals are judicial. In the traditional legal ritual each party purchases the services of a professional gladiator, otherwise known as a divorce attorney. These gladiators arm themselves as heavily as possible and then clash shields on their clients' behalf. One must look over the available options carefully when gladiator shopping, because they come in many shapes and sizes. Some gladiators are satisfied if they unhorse the opponent. Others fight for the pleasure of the kill and love the feeling of standing with one foot on their opponent's chest and driving their blade through the vanquished one's throat. Gladiators with nicknames like "the barracuda" or "the ball-buster" can always be located—or avoided. People generally respond defensively to attack, so both soon-to-be ex-spouses become more and more angry at each other until their hatred is so vehement that they can get over any underlying desire to reunite. The negative consequences of this sort of adversarial ritual are well documented in the records of mental health centers and psychiatric hospitals. Divorce support groups form as a ritual for helping angry people let go of their anger so that they can form new productive relationships. There must be a better way to handle ending a relationship than the traditional legal ritual.

Divorce mediation is a progressive up-and-coming ritual in which benevolent lawyers and therapists work together to help couples negotiate the terms of their divorce in an amicable fashion. The trouble with divorce mediation is that it rests on a new and alien view of human nature, namely, that people may be willing to compromise with each other to avoid shedding blood rather than fight on under a banner sporting the motto "I Win, You Lose." Though helpful, this approach is probably never going to be the prevailing ritual because it only appeals to those who are ready to let go of their mission in the marriage. Why on earth would divorcing people settle for less when they can have it all? Moreover, why let estranged spouses off the hook after years of mistreatment when they can be taught a valuable lesson by taking them for all they're worth—and taking the children as well. Though mediation is a step in the right direction toward benevolent rituals, divorce mediators are among the first to say that mediation is only for certain people.

The limited range of options for divorcing people demonstrates a need for a new generation of positive rituals to help bring closure to marriages that are ending and to encourage divorced people to make a fresh start. This new breed of rituals has shortened the grieving period in broken relationships considerably. Under the current system couples are unlikely to agree to participate in joint rituals, but what if these rituals became as embedded in our lives as weddings and funerals? Admittedly, most of the following suggestions are the untried ideas (although a few have been used) and musings of a frustrated therapist:

1. Why not conduct a divorce ceremony that requires thought, investment of time, and whatever finances are available? Both ex-spouses would be present and would give their rings back to each other. Perhaps there could be two cakes, with the bride on one and the groom on the other. Maybe their children could give them away. How about arranging the guests so that they could sit on the bride's side or the groom's side—or a third side for those intending to stay friends with both of them? The possible rituals are endless. (This idea isn't as strange as it sounds if you consider the bravely festive tone of an old-fashioned New Orleans funeral.) For one divorcing couple, I collaborated with a Unitarian Universalist minister to develop a divorce ceremony. The plan was to hold the ceremony outside in the church's memorial garden, where the ashes of the dead are interred. Part of the service was a burial of the past, symbolized by the burning of the couple's wedding license (or a copy of it) during the service and the scattering of the ashes in the garden.

2. A divorce shower could help people who can't leave a bad marriage because they can't afford it. The gifts would be those household items the newly divorced people need to get started, including furnishings for the bedrooms in both homes for the children. After all, roughly half of all items in the house need to be replaced by one of the divorcing parties or the other.

3. Perhaps a couple could have their rings melted down and then use the metal and stones to make a sculpture for their children. This might be a first task for divorced parents.

4. Perhaps adult or teenage children could be encouraged to develop rituals for their parents in which they help their parents construct a shrine to the past in each parent's house. They could choose a special spot in each house and put photos and remembrances of the family's life together on the shrine. The children could gather at each house and tell stories of the past to memorialize it.

I have sent a few couples on long journeys who were divorced for some time but were still driving each other crazy. They were sent to a particularly high cliff in northern Michigan overlooking Lake Michigan. I gave them directions sealed in an envelope, with instructions on the envelope describing when to open it. They didn't know where they were going or precisely what they were going to do until they got to a certain location and opened the envelope. The couple were asked to agree that they were ready to have their old marriage end. They were then asked to spend time discussing the parts of their relationship that should be discarded and those that should be kept. Once they arrived at the mysterious location, they held hands and threw their wedding rings off the cliff into Lake Michigan, as per the directions in the envelope. (In one case, a spouse who still had a key to the other's house was asked to throw that into the depths of the lake as well.)

In a modification of this ritual, I have sent couples on a tour boat on Lake Superior along the Pictured Rocks National Lakeshore in Michigan. I instructed them to go to the top deck at precisely the halfway point and, while holding hands, to throw their wedding rings into the lake that's so cold and deep that, according to singer/songwriter Gordon Lightfoot, it "never gives up her dead."

I sent another couple on a more costly mission to end their marriage: They spent weeks collecting mementos of painful events in their marriage and writing accounts of marital incidents they wanted to leave in the past. When the mementos and accounts were all collected and the couple had discussed the meaning of each one, they ritualistically burned the items and papers. They then collected the ashes in a jar. They went on a journey to the Florida everglades and deposited the ashes deep in the swamp. Then they rented a car, drove to Key West, and threw their rings into the ocean at a precise location at the moment the sun set. Finally, the divorcing couple walked to the other side of the island; they stayed awake on the beach, contemplating their futures, until the sun rose in the morning. (Although this was an expensive trip, at least the money went to tourism rather than gladiators!)

A simpler version of the aforementioned ritual can be used with less embittered couples, or ones with less money. They can be directed to do the same collecting, writing, and burning but sent on a simpler trip. Often, I send couples or individuals to a virgin white pine forest where there's a log chapel on a hill in a state park. I ask them to sit in the third row of the chapel and contemplate their decision to leave the past behind; if they can both reach this decision, they are to look out from the hill and pick a spot to bury the ashes in an unmarked grave.

Readers may be skeptical about a couple's willingness to perform these rituals. The key to understanding their motivation is to recognize that people will do unusual things when they're in a high level of emotional pain. People who are suffering will do most anything that gives them hope of getting relief. A confident therapist can give them that hope. If therapists keep creating and using rituals for divorce, they may become part of accepted tradition.

Where might this way of thinking lead? Let me conclude with a humorous picture of a couple in business-like clothes standing before a judge, justice, or clergyperson. They return their rings to each other amid ritualized phrases with vows of how they'll work together in their children's best interest. When asked the magic question, each responds, "I don't!" The minister intones, "I now pronounce you man and woman," and they go off to two separate receptions where available people of the opposite sex abound. A bit farfetched? Perhaps, but the way our society's helping people start new lives needs a lot of help.

The need for new and better ways of divorcing is particularly evident in cases where mishandled divorces result in young people becoming assaultive toward their parents. Helping people divorce well will reduce the number of symptomatic adolescents because their explosiveness is often a metaphor for the anger, lack of forgiveness, and intolerance still present in the postdivorce parental relationship. Until we learn to handle divorces more effectively, the task for therapists will continue to be how to help abused parents rally their energies to successfully stop the abuse. In Chapter 5 I will explore methods for motivating abused parents to take action.

FIVE

Getting Abused Parents to Take Action

The greatest roadblock to change is the hopelessness that abused parents feel and the inertia that results from their despair. Parents of aggressive adolescents appear to be either paralyzed into an emotionless stupor or activated to perform a set of ritualized reactions in which they helplessly rage against the tyranny of their children. Some therapists assume that parents of teenagers who are out of control are insecure or inadequate. They assume that parents who appear passive and overwhelmed have always been troubled and conclude that the parents' symptoms explain why their children are abusing them. When they see people acting passively, they assume those parents are passive by nature. What they don't see is how behavior is shaped by relationships, how parents who seem helpless and inept may have become that way because their resources were slowly exhausted as they tried to cope with impossible situations.

It isn't necessarily true that parents asking for help with acting-out teenagers were weak or unsympathetic prior to the problems with their sons or daughters. Their teenagers may have defeated them at every turn as they attempted to assert their parental authority. Often, these parents are caught in a recursive cycle that, like a snowball rolling down a hill, takes on a life of its own. The more their teenagers humiliate them, both privately and publicly, the more hopeless and helpless parents become. Therapists who diagnose these parents as inadequate or blame them for the behavior of their children only perpetuate their powerlessness. These mental health professionals then take the position that the child's behavior is the result of a complicated psychodynamic problem that parents lack the expertise to understand and deal with.

As the picture grows clearer of a society where parents are moved out of the treatment of their children, rather than in, it's obvious why parents who are abused by their children are reluctant to take action to stop the aggression against them. Professionals often communicate to parents that they're in the way and are not up to the task of bringing their children under control.

The approach I discuss in these pages for motivating parents varies quite a bit depending on which parental style the therapist is faced with. Regardless of parental style, therapists must presume that something they can do in relationship to the troubled family holds the key to improving a potentially dangerous situation.

THE APATHETIC PARENT

Parents who appear apathetic when they enter treatment posture themselves like battle-worn veterans of a major war. They face abusiveness and humiliation with a stoic facade that belies the pain they suffer every day. When asked what it is they need help with, these parents describe horrible situations in a manner one would use for a discussion of what color their house should be painted. Their descriptions are recitations of facts accompanied only by a feeling of resignation. Abused parents feel the situation is the only way it can be. Despite feeling horror at the repeated abuse and pain, they become helpless and allow the cycle of fear and abuse to continue, believing that nothing can be done. Therapists and parents facing an abusive adolescent must realize that they're better off taking any reasonable action rather than allowing a terrible situation to continue.

Feelings are spurs to action. For parents afraid to act, feeling becomes dangerous. And so, in addition to being worn out, they're often afraid to feel outraged for fear they'll do something terrible. These abused parents can't find their feelings, so the therapist must lend them his or hers. Parents can be helped to recapture feelings of outrage at their child's provocations: not only hurt and anger for how they've been treated but also sorrow for themselves—which, despite its bad press, is a healthy form of self-respect. The therapist isn't trying to get the parents to express their feelings or achieve any kind of catharsis but is just trying to help them get in touch with the reactions necessary to mobilize actions.

The more the therapist discusses the situation and tries to elicit an emotional reaction from abused parents, the more closed and withholding the parents seem. Therefore, the therapist must project a great deal of emotion on their behalf, namely, astonishment that they have been subjected to such abuse and anger that the abuse continues. When parents are describing their child's abusive behavior, the therapist might respond with, "Your own son speaks to you like that?" or "It's just terrible that you're being treated that way!" If during a family therapy session the son interrupts to angrily defend his actions, the therapist may say, "I'm certain you have important ideas you want to get through to your parents but adults can't hear you when you speak to them like that." The therapist must empathize with parents' anger at the injustice and with the pain they're experiencing. In this way the therapist can begin to break the paralysis that leads parents to accept being mistreated by their children. It might even be necessary to encourage detailed descriptions of the abuse because apathetic parents become so child-focused that they may only report the teenager's complaints about *them!* The therapist should act surprised that other professionals would consider blaming parents for their children's misbehavior and that other therapists would suggest that hospitals know more about helping children than the parents who raised them.

Therapists might see themselves as the family conscience in a situation of parent abuse. Parents must begin to feel angry, hopeful, or excited about the possibility that something can really change. The interview could focus, for example, on what the family will be like after this problem's solved or on how much the parents enjoyed their child before the abusive behavior began. Hopeless people often rewrite the past in a hopeless light, so they may need help remembering the times when they felt competent as parents and when they were proud to show off their son or daughter.

The relationship with a sympathetic but hopeful therapist gives parents strength. By being both understanding and determined, the therapist opens parents' eyes to the realization that everything possible really hasn't been tried. As parents feel understood and begin to believe they can improve their lives, they move naturally toward a willingness to take action. A therapist who pressures abused parents to act usually sees them becoming less and less motivated to do so because they feel criticized for not having taken action before.

The increased presence of any emotion in parents during a therapy session is a sign that the therapy is succeeding in moving them toward a readiness to take some action. Surprisingly, young people at most levels of aggression will begin to settle down as they see their parents becoming more hopeful and determined. Troubled adolescents seem to want their parents to remember what it was like to have self-respect when their children's behavior wasn't the only measure of it. In some families apathy is so entrenched that the therapist must go back to the day their baby was born to find a moment when parents felt hope and love.

CLINICAL VIGNETTE: ANGRY AT THE WORLD

Parents of abusive teenagers often enter treatment angry at the world because of the injustice they've experienced and the world's unresponsiveness. Parents' feelings of injustice are caused by the incredible lack of sympathy they've encountered from other adults while trying to solve their children's problems. Parents are often criticized and humiliated by other adults when they've tried to take charge of their children. Consider Bruce and his father.

Bruce was 17 years old and refused to take any responsibility for helping keep up the house since his mother died 2 years earlier. Bruce continued to expect money for many things and use of the car that his father provided. Whenever his father said no, Bruce became verbally abusive, screaming things like, "You never give me anything anyway. Why should it be any different now?" This barrage of verbal abuse continued until Bruce's father felt he'd had enough; he went on strike (with a therapist's support). Bruce's dad stopped giving him cash, stopped making meals and providing transportation, and said no when Bruce wanted to use the car. He picketed the house with a sign that said FATHER ON STRIKE AGAINST UNGRATEFUL CHILDREN. In order to neutralize his father's increasing control over the household, Bruce went to the parents of friends and told them his father was refusing to feed him. Those parents began a campaign to help the poor fellow. They sent him home with money and bags of groceries and offered him places to live—all without ever contacting Bruce's father to find out if there was any truth to Bruce's claims. Bruce's father at first felt helpless and became despondent; then he decided to contact these freelance social workers to explain the situation, thank them for their kindness, and ask them to stop interfering.

WHO'S REALLY AT FAULT?

It's necessary for the therapist to acknowledge and address the parental anger generated by a society that's unresponsive to people who are being abused by their teenage children. Unfortunately, the field of therapy itself has developed a variety of theories that seem designed to amplify the guilt and blame parents feel. Theories in many schools of thought, including family systems theory, tend to blame the parents for their children's lack of control. Before the advent of family therapy, there were many theories explaining children's problems as the result of errors made by parents. The idea that problems are caused by parents began with a focus on mothers. *Maternal overprotectiveness* was thought to cause many problems of separation in adolescents. A theory also existed that explained schizophrenia as having been caused by a *schizophrenogenic mother*, who specifically trained the adolescent to lose his or her mind. Theories range from those that blame children's problems on "weak" parents who lack parenting skills to those that implicate a schizophrenogenic mother. R. D. Laing once referred to the family as the "concentration camp" of modern society. Even within the family therapy movement there was an undercurrent of parent blaming from the beginning. Early work developed the *double-bind theory* of schizophrenia, which described psychosis as the result of parental communication patterns that produced psychotic symptoms in children. Use of the term *scapegoating* to describe a child's involvement in a marital struggle suggested that parents intentionally encouraged terrible symptoms in their children for selfish reasons.

There are many reasons that therapists develop and believe theories that blame parents. In severely disturbed families, parents are indeed often uncooperative or just plain difficult. They may have been through previous parent-blaming sessions, and they enter therapy already angry. Passive parents who let their children do bad things are easy to dislike; angry ones look like dominating tyrants. Some parents *do* misuse their power to mistreat and abuse children, and it can be difficult to tell which kind of parent a therapist is dealing with. A therapist's ability to tell the difference between truly abusive parents and abused ones who are angry may also depend on whether the parents in a particular case resemble the therapist's own parents and strike a chord of dislike. A reaction toward parents is sure to be emotionally loaded under the best of circumstances, and a reaction of anger can pop up suddenly in any normal adult, even a therapist.

If blame for children's misbehavior is to be assigned, parents could be blamed for feeling guilty for having run out of solutions for what has become a very difficult situation. Any of us could run out of ideas when faced with a tough challenge. Yet professionals slap parents on their wrists for having been poor parents or even malicious ones. The slap on the wrist lowers parents' already questionable status even further and reduces the likelihood they'll go home and take decisive and responsible action to help their children. In fact, these parents are being treated like children themselves.

It's important that the family unit be seen as the source of power when treating teenagers. Whatever the threat, it's best that family members and friends be the people to carry out actions that intervene in aggressive behavior. If a teenager must be restrained when breaking things or picked up and brought home after running away, the effectiveness of the action in bringing about lasting change increases when the people taking action are closely related to the adolescent. If the interventionist is a family member, the young person must concede that things in his or her family are changing and may begin changing in response to the new experience.

There are situations, though, where parents may need additional help to physically manage a teenager who threatens harm or runs away from home. When all other avenues have failed or people simply can't be found to help manage threats, it's appropriate to have families turn to the authorities. One option for legal action is to file a petition with the juvenile court; usually this takes the form of some kind of truancy or incorrigibility charge. Unfortunately, experience has demonstrated that these steps often aren't acted on by the court. Even if a petition is followed up properly by the court, it may take 6 months in some jurisdictions for an adolescent to be called in for a preliminary hearing. Therefore, in most cases the juvenile court shouldn't be relied on unless a criminal charge, such as assault, can be pursued. Once adjudicated for incorrigibility and found guilty, a young person often discovers that violation of the conditions of probation will not result in further consequences. The court seems to be more effective when a young person commits a genuine crime; then, decisive legal action allows children to see that other adults feel the same way their parents do about their behavior and that those others are willing to act in concert with the parents.

Police may be called in an emergency, but it's critical that therapists know how the police force in each community responds to adolescent domestic problems. The police in some cities either won't respond or will send someone out to speak nicely to the teenager and parents. If reasoning doesn't work, these police may act as if there's nothing else they can do unless an actual assault has occurred. However, some police departments understand that they're a sign of power with teenagers, and they take forceful measures to assist parents.

In one such case a therapeutic response was achieved by calling the police. A 14-year-old boy threatened to kill his mother with a ball-peen hammer. He had the hammer in his hand and was moving toward her while screaming threats and obscenities about how she was running his life. She managed to call the local police, who sent out an officer (whom she later described as being the size of former Chicago Bears linebacker Dick Butkus). When the officer, who tried talking to the young fellow in his room, said something disagreeable to him about listening to his mother, the teenager said, "Fuck you, pig!" The therapist, who already knew that police in this town didn't always play by the rules, wasn't surprised to hear that the officer then grabbed the shocked young man by the front of his shirt. According to the boy's mother the officer said, "Don't you ever speak to me that way again, and I don't want to hear that you ever speak to your mother that way again, either. If I hear that you threaten her I'll be back, and you won't like what'll happen!" The officer then reportedly let go of the boy with a jerk, without harm. Very few additional therapy sessions were needed once the teenager understood there were powers greater than himself that would come forward on his mother's behalf. Although the police were helpful in this case, a relative is a better choice than a police officer because a relative cares about the teenager, is more predictable than the police, and will be seen by the adolescent as a permanent ongoing resource. An officer's influence is lost as soon as the adolescent realizes that the individual's availability is limited by job demands. Calling the police can also be risky: If an officer is called and then fails to take decisive action, the outcome is worse than if he had never been summoned. The teenager then knows that the result of the ongoing threat to call police is inconsequential, and this leaves parents looking more impotent than ever.

The plight of abused parents is further complicated by the fact that the police department often doesn't take adolescents' threats or attacks on their parents seriously. Many departments won't come out on such calls because adolescent struggles are domestic in nature. The courts often won't take legal action against young people because criminal activity against parents isn't considered a crime. A young person who steals a parent's car is seen as acting out rather than as a car thief. An adolescent who is caught in this act by the police is usually taken home to be disciplined by his or her parents rather than put in a holding cell pending charges for auto theft. Children who physically attack their parents don't necessarily get charged with assault and battery. Adolescents' crimes only seem to become crimes when they're perpetrated against someone outside the family

The difficulty getting outside help makes it harder for parents who already feel overwhelmed to rise up and take action. Even other parents are likely to say, "So why do you let him do that?" rather than, "You are clearly being victimized by your son."

In many cases the therapist's role may be more that of an advocate for the parents than a therapist. The power of a therapist who can communicate the message that parents are being abused can influence other professionals to help. Actions taken as an advocate may succeed in getting new rights for parents. For instance, parents often won't fight back against or restrain their teenagers in any way when being assaulted because of the threat of legal action against them, but a therapist who's willing to support parents by documenting the difference between abuse and restraint can emotionally free them to take action. Therapists who make it clear that they will go to court, write letters, and support the use of restraint, when appropriate, can help get parents out of a position where they feel helpless and without recourse.

A second reason parents hesitate to take action against their adolescent is the fear of initiating a violent incident. A mother may be frightened that an argument between her husband and son will escalate into violence and that someone will really get hurt. A mother may be faced with a young man who's bigger and stronger than she is. Parents who were abused as children may become immobilized by fear when anyone, including their own child, threatens them.

Although it's hard to describe, there's a frame of mind that parents can attain that will usually make it unnecessary for them to physically wrestle their child to the ground. This mind-set is an attitude of parental indignation and determination to stand up for the right to act like a parent. It includes a willingness to take charge and solve the problem no matter what it takes. This mind-set is the difference between wrestling with one's child to keep him or her from leaving against one's will versus standing in the doorway with a hand on each door jamb and saying, "You may not leave!" with a conviction that communicates that one means it. In the latter case the adolescent has a difficult decision to make: To get out the door he or she must actively overpower a parent who isn't attacking in any way.

If parents stand up for their rights and restrain out-of-control children when it's necessary, the therapist can get right on the phone to the child protective services worker. In most cases after a phone conversation with a therapist who explains the situation, professionals such as social workers, school personnel, and clergy relax and stop challenging the appropriateness of parents' actions. A family therapy session that includes a social service worker who clarifies what parents may and may not do can also free up parents to take calm and decisive action.

Therapists take it upon themselves to intervene in a defective process of support for parents. They agree to take some risk in situations that are growing progressively more dangerous because troubled families that remain unchanged will get more and more out of control. Is it risky helping parents to take action? Sure it is. But the risk is greater if therapists are passive or if they overreact to dangerous situations in ways that may break up or ruin families. One can only hope that when the prosecuting attorney asks the therapist on the witness stand what he or she did to try to prevent a disaster, the therapist has a better explanation than "I worked on helping them communicate."

CLINICAL VIGNETTE: THE CHANGELING

David was 16 years old. He and his family had moved from Chapel Hill to the rural part of North Carolina I was working in. David was brought for therapy after having been released from the local juvenile detention facility. David had served 6 months there after breaking into a dry cleaning store and stealing money. His release was provisional and could be revoked at any time. Although most therapy sessions were with David, his mother, and his stepfather, occasionally sessions were with David alone.

David was a tall, fair-skinned, blonde boy who could speak very well for himself—or act like a streetwise thug. His mother, Mrs. Gilchrist, was frail looking despite her powerful voice. Mr. Gilchrist was tall, broad-shouldered, and balding; his gentle voice was surprising in someone so large and macho looking. Throughout the first seven sessions, therapy went through a process of improvements and relapses. At home the situation would swing back and forth from a fairly affectionate relationship between David and his mother to a conflictual one, where she would scream at him for hours on end. Such turbulent times would often land Mrs. Gilchrist in the hospital with her blood sugar raging out of control or her blood pressure escalating dangerously. Mrs. Gilchrist got along with her husband of 2 years when things were going smoothly in her relationship with David, but she had terrible conflict with Mr. Gilchrist when David was struggling with her.

When I talked to him alone, David was usually fairly cooperative. He demonstrated a good heart by speaking in a genuinely concerned way about his mother and really seemed to want to do well and stay out of the detention center. He accepted his stepfather in the family and had most of his conflict with his mother. Since David's biological father had left when he was born and was never heard from again, David didn't seem to experience any loyalty conflict as a result of liking his stepfather.

After I became frustrated by yet another relapse in the Gilchrist family, in which Mrs. Gilchrist was again screaming bitterly about David's lack of concern for her, I decided it was time to take a bigger step. Since Cloé Madanes was coming to our institute to do some live supervision, I scheduled my session with the Gilchrist family so that Cloé could observe us from behind the one-way mirror. Cloé had a telephone link to me enabling her to call into the room and make suggestions or observations. We agreed that rather than implement a specific strategy for change I would begin the session by exploring the current relationships—it was always an adventure to see who would be loving or enraged toward whom in this family.

I pursued a course of interview that would clarify what progress had been made in the therapy to date. The session began with both parents talking about how much better David was doing. Their description of him as cooperative and more present in the family reminded me of previous "improvements," in which David would behave better as long as they didn't push him too hard. I decided that pushing him would be a good way to see if he really had made progress and could accept authority being exercised over him.

The following transcript excerpt illustrates how a clinician using a destabilizing therapy increases the pressure in order to get people ready to change (as opposed to the activity of a clinician using a stabilizing therapy, who calms things down on a weekly basis). Sometimes it takes a significant increase in discomfort to help complacent or depressed parents take action.

"On the one hand, that all sounds really great, but it also sounds familiar." I began in response to the parents' praise of David. "We've been along this route about three times since the four of us have been meeting together, where things suddenly start looking better—"

Mrs. Gilchrist talked over my last few words to insist, "He's never done this good since, well, in the past 3 years, I'd say."

"I remember a period right after we met with the probation officer and he got in trouble again and was in court, when you were describing it pretty much the same," I continued.

Mr. Gilchrist explained, "The only thing different now is we've been talking here—"

He was anxiously interrupted by his wife saying, "He comes in, sits down, and talks with us."

Mr. Gilchrist added, "We didn't have that before."

As they spoke David was sitting slouched down in his chair, legs stretched out, arms crossed tightly, his head tilted forward until his chin was on his chest. He wasn't saying anything, but his silence was hard and heavy. It seemed to me that his parents' deflection of any discussion of his potential to do badly was too insistent and sounded a bit frightened. This is often the case when families are walking on eggshells around adolescents who they're afraid might blow up if pushed. To find out whether David really had better self-control, I decided to keep pushing until I myself saw signs of improvement in David that were consistent with the description being presented of him by Mr. and Mrs. Gilchrist. Cloé called into the interview room to suggest that a way to get the family beyond pretending that things were okay would be to discuss the future and talk about what it would be like the next time David got arrested. If things are truly improved, I reasoned, we should find ourselves having a calm conversation; if David was still troubled, the family should begin to act the way they acted when they were mad at him.

"On the one hand, I think that's great," I said. "On the other hand, David has been so persistent in getting himself back into trouble that I think we have to take a serious look at the future. We need to at least discuss the possibility that David could do something serious before too long."

Mr. Gilchrist responded immediately with, "Yeah, I know, it's the track record." His agreement was followed by an eruption of everyone in the room talking at once.

David was becoming more sullen during this conversation, so I addressed his confusion over the discussion. "I want to be as hopeful as possible for you, David, and I want to be as hopeful as possible for your family, but I also feel an obligation to help you really be prepared for it if the bottom falls out again."

Mrs. Gilchrist continued to take her extreme position of defending him with the same gusto she showed when screaming at him during bad moments: "I don't know. It's the first time I've ever seen him change like he has, you know. I sat down and talked to him today. He said, 'Mom I'm only 16 years old.' He said, 'It's time for me to take control of my life.' And that's the first time he's ever said that to me, and he's going back to work on the 16th, through the school system. And, um, I don't know if he's still smoking pot or not. I haven't caught him, and I haven't seen it. It was about 3 weeks ago; last time I found it I threw it away. So I don't know if he's still doing it. It could be, he's on the street, you know. As far as I know, I don't think he is."

Mrs. Gilchrist went on to talk about other things that worried her, things that would make any parent uncertain about how well a child was doing. Among these was a recent incident in which David was picked up and taken to the police station while carrying a barbecue grill down the street after hours. He claimed he had found the grill, but everyone involved was a bit skeptical.

I continued, "Now this sounds familiar. Curfew violation alone is enough to get him sent back to detention because he's on temporary release rather than probation."

Mrs. Gilchrist replied, "Well, he went to see the juvenile officer Tuesday, and he says it's nothing. And I talked to his probation officer, and he says it's nothing as long as they don't charge him with the theft of the barbecue grill."

I punctuated, "*If* they don't."

She continued, "I just want to say this is one time I believe him because I said, 'David, if you did steal it, just tell me, maybe I can go to the people.' "

The point that David was still doing some of the troubled things he used to do had been made. Mrs. Gilchrist continued to defend him until I changed the subject. Mrs. Gilchrist had been working extremely long hours for a person with her medical problems. Her long hours and the physical nature of her work (stocking shelves) had contributed to many hospitalizations. I'd encouraged Mrs. Gilchrist to consider applying for disability or to find some way to work less, but she hadn't followed through on my suggestions. I'd often wondered what the relationship was between David's acting out and his mother's poor self-care and decided that this was a good time to try to discover it. Leaning toward Mrs. Gilchrist I began, "Let me ask you: What's happened with your situation as far as work? You were working a lot of hours, and then you had to stop working because of your health."

She answered, "Well, I tried to go back to work, but I had to quit because it didn't work out. I couldn't handle it."

I began to wonder if David was doing better at home because his mother had finally accepted her limitations and stopped working. I pushed the connection between her illness and David's symptoms to see if Mrs. Gilchrist would accept or fight against the idea. "You know, I've seen that when you're working yourself to death, at those same times David's destroying himself out on the streets. He's getting into drugs and fights, and he's got people trying to kill him. If you can really stick with it and set an example for David of knowing your limits and taking proper care of yourself, maybe David can control himself, too. Let's assume for a moment that you got really tired of being at home, okay, and you just felt cooped up in the house and you were just getting fried, and you said, 'I've got to go back to work,' and you went back."

She laughed, "That's what I just did."

Mrs. Gilchrist would begin taking care of herself, then swing back to overworking until she couldn't stand it, then begin doing better again. Simultaneously, David moved in and out of being a delightful young man and acting like a punk. The connection had been made between David's self-destructiveness and that of his mother. I left the connection between David's problems and those of his mother for then, intending to come back to the subject later if information continued to support the validity of the connection. Because David looked so uninterested in this conversation, I began talking to him and discussing his progress. This should have been a reasonable and encouraging conversation if he were doing as well as his parents had claimed. "You know, David," I began, "your parents are suggesting you're seeing things differently lately. Do you think you have a new, healthier, outlook on accepting the rules and not getting in trouble with the law?"

David responded lethargically saying, "I don't know. I'm screwing up a little bit."

"What's your opinion now about violating the law, about stealing, about doing drugs?"

With David on the spot, his mother tried to talk over him, but he could still be heard to mumble, "I don't care."

Surprised, I answered, "You don't care about it?"

David broke in, "I didn't say that, man; I said that laws is wrong, but I don't think smoking pot's too wrong. I don't even drink, man, because I don't like drinking, either. All I do is smoke pot. Not too many people that can make me stop doing that."

David was using a snotty tone of voice when I asked him about his attitudes toward the law and misbehavior, so I tried another approach—focusing on his plans for the future. A young person with plans for the future is more likely to keep himself under control than one who can only focus on what he's feeling today. "David, what are you thinking of doing with yourself in the next 5 years? You're almost 16, aren't you?"

His mother answered, "Two weeks from today, in fact."

I continued, "Being 16 has its good points and its bad ones. You're reaching an age when your decisions are more your own. You're approaching 18 fast. What are you thinking of doing then?"

David answered sullenly, "I don't know."

"Do you plan to finish high school?"

"Yeah."

"What happened with this year? Were you able to finish it?"

"I finished, but I failed."

"So you're going to have to repeat the grade?"

"Yeah."

I began to address the future again and asked, "David, when you finish high school what are you thinking of doing?"

He replied, "I don't know. Probably going to go into construction."

I prodded, "Get into construction?"

He answered, "Home construction."

Hoping we had a lead on an identifiable future, I said, "Yeah? That's great. You pretty handy with a hammer?"

Unfortunately, he answered, "I don't know. I don't even know why I have it in mind. I just take every day as it comes. I could be dead tomorrow, man." I tried to respond, but he went on, "Man, I don't give a fuck about tomorrow."

We went on to discuss the future. We explored the possibility of David's going into the military, but he showed about the same amount of enthusiasm for that possibility as he had demonstrated in discussing home construction. Mr. Gilchrist got involved in the conversation for the first time that session. He had been in the Marines and recommended the Air Force. He was leaning forward in his chair and seemed to have a burning need to be useful to David. Again I was hopeful that we might have a lead we could capitalize on by getting David and his family interested in something together. As with every attempt thus far, this one also fell flat:

"So, David," I said, "you'd been talking with your folks about the military."

"Not really," he answered. That ended that.

Having failed with this line of questioning, I picked up where I'd left off earlier. I turned to Mr. and Mrs. Gilchrist and said, "You know, considering the way David's reacting and how little he's thinking ahead, you two ought to be considering the fact that he may very well go out and do something more. David, I appreciate your optimism but—"

David interrupted and in a nasty tone snapped, "I just don't like being here is what I'm not acting right for, okay? That's why I'm not acting right. I don't like being here! I want to leave, go home."

Cloé called in and described a way to defuse such an escalation. She suggested that I define David's outburst as proof that what I was saying was correct. That way, since any further blowups on his part would reinforce my argument, he would probably calm down.

"This reaction is exactly what we're talking about," I pointed out. "All we did was increase his anxiety a little, put a little pressure on him with what we're talking about today, and he's starting to lash out."

His mother responded weakly, "He didn't want to come this morning. I had to threaten and everything else to get him up this morning."

On the one hand, my hypothesis that David's improvement was artificial and unreliable was being supported. On the other hand, like his parents, I hated to upset the applecart and make trouble where there didn't appear to be any. After an internal struggle over whether to continue the plan to push the family, I got beyond my feelings and continued with my intention to keep showing the need for vigilance and action on the part of David's parents. I continued focusing on future problems: "I'm afraid David's still got a view of life that sets him up to get in trouble again. What I'd like to do is ask you to think ahead into the future. Assume for a moment—we're just assuming for a moment here, David—that David gets himself arrested. Let's say he goes to the police station. What happens then? You get a call?"

Mrs. Gilchrist sullenly responded, "Uh-huh."

"And then of course they'd be saying they want you down there, I assume."

"Uh-huh."

"Would both of you go?"

"We both went there the other night," Mrs. Gilchrist answered, referring to the trip to the police station to deal with the barbecue grill incident. The reality of the risk in David's future was beginning to set in. His parents were beginning to reference incidents that could indicate future problems.

"What would happen when you're at the police station?"

Mrs. Gilchrist finally began to tear up and said, "It hurts. You know, what can you do? He's there and you got to go get him. If the offense is bad enough, they take him right to juvenile."

Again using the opportunity Mrs. Gilchrist had offered to frame the future as having serious dangers, I said, "Let's assume it's bad enough for a minute, okay? You mentioned he was hurt last time he went to juvenile detention."

David finally spoke up, saying, "I got in a fight with a kid. He was trying to tell me to do things and I told him no, I'm not going to do them."

I asked, "Are we talking about homosexual stuff here?"

He answered, "Homosexual in a juvenile home? He was telling me to fill up the milk pitcher and clean off his table and stuff like that. I told him to get screwed."

I went on to discuss details of what it would be like on that evening if he were arrested. We discussed bail and whether he could come home. I suggested that if it were a serious crime, he could wind up at a long-term placement such as the Boys' Training School. I walked the parents through the experience of meeting at the juvenile detention program and then going home without him. The mood in the room had become more like that of a funeral, in contrast to the original sense of well-being and complacency.

Mr. Gilchrist echoed the risk of serious charges by adding, "He has five charges. The next one—"

Mrs. Gilchrist broke in, "If he does anything now . . . " Her voice trailed off sounding forlorn.

David began to argue about the details of how the bond would be set and how he'd be just like everyone else and wouldn't be treated differently. His irritated response seemed to be a reaction to his mother's becoming upset. As she began to feel more frightened and aware of the risks of David's getting into more trouble, he began to anticipate her blowing up at him again and getting herself so worked up that she might wind up back in the hospital. David was becoming irritated and was fidgeting in his chair. Trying to calm the mood in the room he began to speak more reasonably. He reassured his mother, saying, "It ain't going to happen, though."

The strategy of being pessimistic was finally bringing David to a more rational posture. His parents no longer seemed like pushovers. As unnatural as it seems, to continue the progress I had to keep speaking pessimistically. "Well, David, I hope you're right," I said. "But the way things have gone, I think your parents have the right to look at the possibilities so they don't get blown away like they have before."

Although David was speaking in an angry tone, he continued to be reassuring, saying, "They ain't going to get blown away. They knew what was coming last time. I was giving them a lot of trouble. They knew it."

As I stuck to the plan, the family began looking more and more as they did when they first started this course of therapy. (David was also cooperative then, when the family began treatment.) The pretense that everything was going fine was dissolving. I persisted in my pessimism, saying, "If David were sure he wasn't going to get in any more trouble, he wouldn't be getting upset about us discussing it. Considering his record, wouldn't you say he'd be likely to get some time in detention?"

Mrs. Gilchrist answered, "If he does something wrong, yeah. They'll keep him till he's 19. They done told him that. He tries to tell me 6 months."

David came back with, "You guys don't even know what you're saying."

"All I know is they told me if you went back, you'd stay till you're 19," Mrs. Gilchrist responded angrily.

David finally pulled his trump card and emphatically said, "Let's just go. This is the last time I'm coming here, anyways."

Ignoring his demand, I continued, "I don't want to stop quite there. Let's go a little further and take a look, okay? In 2 weeks he's going to be 16, and in North Carolina if he does something serious once he's 16, they could choose to try him as an adult. So we might be talking state prison. Those prison veterans are known to be pretty rough on new guys, especially young ones."

"They might get a big surprise," David said quietly.

Mrs. Gilchrist abruptly changed the subject, saying, "He's sort of upset. The people that lived in the apartment next to us, they took their kids the other day 'cause the father, the uncle, and I guess no telling how many others was having sex with their little girls, 8- and 9-year-old little girls. And we were hearing it, but we didn't know what we were hearing. And they took the kids, and David wants to kill the father."

I added, "And the scary part is that in prison they're especially rough on young guys who mistreat their mothers. Motherhood is a big thing in this country. Young guys like that are second on the list to child molesters, and child molesters have to be put in a special wing in the state prison because the guys will kill them. So, David, you could wind up in state prison, and you'd have a lot of new experiences by the time you got out."

David began to defend himself more appropriately. He began reporting data on his record rather than having emotional outbursts. "Ma, tell him what Mr. Moore said. My name hasn't come up over the last 2 months. My name hasn't been mentioned in anything."

I reply, "Two months is a good start, but we're talking a couple years for you to be clean."

"Yeah, but still, man. I don't want to hear it."

The family's distress had increased dramatically since the beginning of the session. Distress is an essential ingredient in the recipe for motivation. With many families, discomfort must be cultivated before family members can be directed to take steps for bringing about change. Without first having their discomfort nurtured, people may not be feeling an urgent need to get out of their unfortunate situation. The Gilchrists' distress had grown until it was sufficient for them to begin intervening in the cycle, which was now heading toward a relapse. I began making a connection between David's of mishandling his life and his mother's mishandling of her illnesses.

I began by speaking with Mrs. Gilchrist. "When David got into trouble and was placed in juvenile detention, things got very rough at home. Mrs. Gilchrist, you were upset almost all the time, and you were having a lot of medical problems from the stress. You were hospitalized a couple times for your asthma, and you were screaming and yelling a lot." Then I turned to Mr. Gilchrist and said, "Do you think your wife will really avoid getting back into slowly killing herself if David decides he's going to risk his life and slowly kill himself?"

Mr. Gilchrist replied, "I don't know. Lately she just figures the same way I do. If he's bound and determined to get into problems, there's nothing you can do."

David's posture had changed, and he was looking at whoever was speaking in an interested way. Mr. and Mrs. Gilchrist were both leaning forward in their chairs. I took this change in manner to mean I was on the right track. I told Mrs. Gilchrist, "You know, it may be that David's taking care of himself and has stopped slowly destroying himself because you have."

Without hesitation she said, "Could be. He's upset because I went back to work. He told me, 'You don't need to work.' Doctor didn't even want to pass me for the physical for the job, and I begged him. I told him, I said, 'I've got to go to work. I need the money bad, you know.'"

David again began participating in a more interested way, without any sign of a hostile attitude: "I haven't asked her for money in a long time, either."

His mother responded with, "No. He knows we don't have it, so he don't ask for it."

This admission that David had done better when his mother wasn't working gave me a great opportunity to stress the connection between Mrs. Gilchrist's mistreatment of herself and David's misbehavior. Of course, I wanted to make sure that Mrs. Gilchrist had a source of income before I encouraged her to give up working. I continued, "And when you were killing yourself, he was demanding a huge amount of money. If you were to stop working so hard once and for all, could you collect disability?"

She answered, "I am drawing Social Security."

"Okay. So there's some money coming in."

"Oh, yeah. We get a little behind, but it ain't too bad."

Mrs. Gilchrist's admission about the family's financial needs opened up the possibility that David could be encouraged to do well and stay free in order to help her. "Social Security's still a very limited income," I said. "David, I wonder what your plans are for helping support your mom. You'll be working this summer, I understand. How much do you think you'll be making?"

He immediately answered, "About $100 a week."

"David, I think your mom's going to need your help in order to see to it she doesn't wind up having to go back to work. What would you think about giving about 50 of that to your mom to help her?"

He responded, "I gave her money every week when I worked last summer, too. I already know that kind of stuff."

A little surprised by his compassionate statement, I said, "That's great. If you make some clear plans for the future, you may be able to make a good enough income that your mom will know she'll have a comfortable future. I'm a parent, too, and one of the things that we parents count on is that our kids are going to be there to support us in our old age. I look at my 2-year-old every now and then and say, 'Just remember, Josh, a condo in Florida.' I see now that you think that's important, too. Now you've got to make some plans for the future. Is that something you're willing to do?"

He answered, "Yeah, it is."

I took a break to consult with Cloé behind the one-way mirror. Cloé emphasized the need to be direct with David's mother. Mrs. Gilchrist had demonstrated that she could handle taking responsibility for how her behavior affected her son and that she wasn't experiencing it as blame. Both David and his mother seemed to act more maturely when the connection between their irresponsibilities was being discussed and Mrs. Gilchrist was able to see her son's misbehavior as a way of trying to get help for her by emphasizing a problem.

The parents' attitude in this session had moved from complacent denial to outrage and struggle with their child and, finally, to compassionate understanding of adolescent behavior they could no longer tolerate or subtly encourage. When we discussed whether David's behavior warranted them feeling complacent, neither he nor his parents could find sufficient evidence to support such a response. Mr. and Mrs. Gilchrist had trouble maintaining a position of outrage because David was basically a nice fellow who was concerned about his mother and willingly gave her a portion of his paychecks to make life easier for her. The final part of the session was spent making David's benevolence explicit and then clearly connecting his concern for his mother to his misbehavior. David's good heart was leading him to ruin and his mother had to be influenced to stop him from sacrificing himself this way. Cloé suggested we frame the discussion in terms of self-respect.

"The most important element everyone must have in order to be successful is self-respect," I said. "David doesn't do things that a guy with enough self-respect would do. And Mrs. Gilchrist, the way you respond to anxiety, you don't treat yourself respectfully either and you don't take care of yourself."

Mrs. Gilchrist nodded and said, "Yeah."

I continued, "David needs to see you find other ways of supporting yourself besides working yourself to death. Take care of your health. Get some activity. Smile more. I don't see you smile here very often. I hate to think it's just me, but I get the feeling that smiling's not something you do very much at home, either."

Mrs. Gilchrist was nodding as I spoke, and David was watching his mother closely. Her positive nonverbal cues showed me I was on the right track, and David's interest supported my confidence in the strategy we'd pursued. Without these positive signs I would have been worried about Mrs. Gilchrist feeling blamed and scolded. "The bottom line is, David loves you so much that when he sees you responding to the anxiety in your life by destroying yourself and he thinks about the possibility of losing you, he just gets nuts."

Mrs. Gilchrist's voice became shaky, and her eyes were wet as she said, "Oh, I know that. Everything would be going good until I got sick and had to go to the hospital. And as soon as I go in the hospital, he'd start getting in trouble in school. I've known that for a long time."

I was a relieved therapist. Because Mrs. Gilchrist had accepted the connection between David's self-destructiveness and hers, I could proceed to validate the connection between them and then direct the session toward an important change. I spoke to Mrs. Gilchrist first: "So your obligation is to continue setting an example for David, an example of someone who has respect for her body. You know, Mr. Gilchrist, I think you could help your wife remember to set a good example."

Sounding very sincere, he answered, "Yeah, I'll try to take care of myself better, too."

I leaned toward Mrs. Gilchrist and said, "I'd like you to thank your son for being so concerned. I'd like you to tell him—"

She interrupted and said, "Thanks." David gave a big smile and sat up in his chair.

I said, "Tell him you appreciate his help."

"He knows I do."

"He needs to hear it clearly: 'David, I appreciate that you love me so much that you would hurt yourself to help me.' "

"He knows that," she said, again avoiding a direct response.

"And I'd like you to promise him that you're going to take good care of yourself and that he won't have to do that again."

"Okay, I will."

"Tell him clearly. I want him to hear every word."

"I'll take care of myself if you won't get in no more trouble."

I continued to prompt, "It's not a deal. I just want you to say, 'David, I promise I'm going to take good care of myself and care of my body, and you're never going to have to do that again.'"

Mrs. Gilchrist finally said, "I'll take care of myself so you won't have to do that again, okay?"

David nodded, and I told her, "Now give him a hug and a kiss."

Mrs. Gilchrist put out her arms to David and said, "Give me a hug." David immediately leaned forward and hugged and kissed his mom and even lingered a bit.

Finally, I ratified the agreement and included Mr. Gilchrist by stating, "This is a great example of how you can help the people you love most by helping yourselves and by really taking care of yourselves. What I'd like you to do is each put a hand out right here." At Cloé's suggestion I had mother, stepfather, and son put one hand on top of each other's, like football players coming out of a huddle. "One for all and all for one, okay? I can tell that you're a family that really love and care about each other and that you don't want David being off somewhere instead of with you."

With tears running down her cheeks, Mrs. Gilchrist nudged David with her foot and said, "You know that, don't you?"

"Yeah, I know that," he answered.

When the session ended, the hierarchy had been corrected despite having a mother apologize to her son. Mr. Gilchrist was leaning toward his wife and was holding and stroking her hand for the first time that session. David was playfully nudging his mother with his feet, and everyone was smiling, including me.

Mrs. Gilchrist came in alone for the next session and reported that David was acting up. As we discussed the situation, I learned Mrs. Gilchrist had begun bleeding from the rectum several days earlier and hadn't gone to the doctor. I insisted that she go home, apologize to David for breaking her promise to take care of herself, and go to the doctor; when she got home from the doctor, she was to make sure David knew she'd been there.

I met with the family for several more sessions, during which I helped David clearly move into the role of helpful son by describing him that way and encouraging his kind acts. Mr. Gilchrist left the family for about a year, and during that time I encouraged Mrs. Gilchrist to let David take her out to dinner, movies, and other activities while she got used to being without a spouse. According to a 2-year follow-up interview, David stayed out of trouble with the law throughout the remainder of his adolescence.

It's difficult for many therapists to push families as hard as they need to be pushed. Generating a therapeutic level of tension often requires going against the people the therapist is there to help. Creating that tension may even require that the therapist send a family out the door so angry with him or her that they may never come back. To quote Phil McPeek, a friend of mine and early supervisor, "You can't treat anyone unless you're willing to let them walk."

Motivated parents give their therapist more information; discouraged parents answer questions with generalities, which aren't helpful to a therapist who's trying to make a proper assessment. Having successfully motivated parents toward a productive discussion, the therapist must understand how to use the resulting information to identify the level of aggression a family is dealing with and to plan a strategy for change. In the next chapter is a comprehensive set of guidelines for assessing aggression in adolescents and choosing the right strategies for change.

How to Break the Cycle of Intimidation

Most therapists are schooled in a specific approach to treatment. One problem with having a single approach is that the therapist tends to apply that approach in a repetitive and formulaic way regardless of the needs in a particular case (Haley, 1976). This problem is especially pronounced in dealing with an aggressive adolescent, who may trigger an emotional response in the therapist that makes him or her assume immediately that the adolescent is dangerous and malicious. After all, what do most people conclude when faced with open hostility?

When open hostility is mixed with a formulaic approach to treatment, the result is a knee-jerk diagnosis of "bad." The unique details of a case are hard to see when anger, fear, and distaste compromise the therapist's ability to think clearly. It's hard to tell, for example, if a teenage boy who's swearing at his parents is trying to dominate everyone or to get his parents to take charge of a family that's out of control.

In this chapter a framework is presented for assessing motivation and aggression in teenagers and young adults and for guiding the professional in choosing the right strategies to help clients change. The interventions described are by no means exhaustive. These interventions are divided into categories, with examples included. General guidelines based on categories always seem to overlap, so I have to leave it to the reader to adapt these approaches to each new case encountered.

Making distinctions between the various sorts of aggressiveness is the key to treating adolescents properly. Without accurate distinctions the therapist would try to do exactly the same thing to help every client. There are many different kinds of aggression in adolescents, just as there are many differences among them with respect to any trait, so it's critical that the therapist look closely at each young person and his or her family. Seeing the unique characteristics of the young person and family allows the therapist to use a creative approach to look at a wide range of possible interventions.

Many young people who become abusive walk a fine line between threatening violence against their families and actually carrying those threats out. The types of abuse can be grouped into six categories that describe the form of the threat. The accurate placement of a particular adolescent on this continuum depends upon the degree to which the young person has actually engaged in violence and assaultive behavior.

THE LEVELS OF ADOLESCENT AGGRESSION

Level 1: The Petulant Child

Adolescents become enraged when challenged. Their voices rise and they take up an accusatory or pained tone. These teenagers appear so tormented that parents hate to see them in such pain and are likely to give in to a demand or back off from a limit they're trying to set. Level 1 aggression occurred when 13-year-old Matthew, who was reminded angrily and for the 11th time by his father to clean his room, began moaning, "I hate myself. I always do stupid things."

Level 2: A Flair for the Dramatic

Adolescents swear and call their parents names while in a rage. This verbally assaultive behavior implies to many parents that their child is on the verge of violence. It's remarkable how threatening a young person can be; their dramatics often convince parents, who are intimidated by their newly adult-sized kids, that they have something to fear. When 14-year-old Brittany stepped toward her mother and called her a bitch, she was demonstrating Level 2 behavior. If she had added, "Leave me alone, or I'll scratch your eyes out," that behavior would have been Level 3.

Level 3: The Beginning of Damage

Level 3 includes threats to kill or injure parents, siblings, and animals. For this level to be assessed, the young person must never have truly injured any living thing. He or she may have engaged in aggressive acts that caused minimal damage to things that weren't terribly valuable. It's clear at this level that the teenager thinks about how far he or she is going. For instance, 13-year-old Emily might throw a book at the wall but avoids throwing knives or glassware, proving that she is still thinking about how serious the consequences of an action might be.

Level 4: Threatening Gestures and Serious Damage to Possessions

Adolescents at Level 4 actively attack objects. They may knock holes in walls, throw and break valuable objects, or smash windows. Parents who aren't intimidated by the threats at Level 3 usually quail before such an onslaught of aggression. At this level most parents conclude that they have a dangerous child on their hands. The child may threaten to hit a family member with a weapon, such as a hammer or other heavy object, but makes no actual contact. A Level 4 teenager may threaten with a knife but keeps a large distance from the target person and backs off when approached. Young people who move toward an intended victim with a knife are displaying a higher form of aggression than Level 4. It may or may not be wise to get into a struggle with a teenager who's at Level 4 (depending on variables that will be discussed later in this chapter).

Level 5: People Get Hurt

At Level 5, actual violence accompanies threats. Such behavior includes pushing, shouldering, hitting siblings (without serious injury), and doing minor harm to people by throwing objects at them. If they weren't intimidated at earlier levels, parents become frightened at this point because their child is demonstrating that he or she might truly lose control and hurt someone. Nevertheless, injury at this level is minor, and any injury done tends to be incidental. For instance, a boy might throw a stool across a room and hit his sister, who is unexpectedly walking through the door and winds up in harm's way. Even if the stool breaks the sister's arm, the injury is considered unintentional inasmuch as the boy didn't know she was going to step into the room. At Level 5 it's important to determine whether the adolescent made a choice to injure someone or caused the injury as an accidental side effect of the outburst. As long as the injury is unintentional, the young adult is considered to be still in control of the level of force being used.

Level 6: Serious Danger and Harm

Adolescents at Level 6 begin demonstrating dangerous violent behavior. They may begin striking with objects or fists in ways that clearly intend injury or may push someone when it could cause a serious fall. The deliberate use of weapons to cause injury also falls into this category. When 12-year-old Mark hit his brother with a baseball bat, that was Level 6 behavior. However, when 13-year-old Sean picked up a hammer and told his mother he was going to hit her in the head, that wasn't Level 6: Sean's behavior would still be properly assessed as Level 4 because he was threatening with a weapon but without making any contact. The weapon was part of a gesture rather than an attack.

SOME GENERAL PRINCIPLES

♦ Escalation of violence is an interactive process. When parents or others overreact and intervene emotionally, they can cause the adolescent's aggression to escalate to a higher level. Screaming at an already irate teenager is looking for trouble.

♦ Parents must be helped to recognize the difference between words and behaviors that are harmful and those that are just mean and inflammatory. Threats from adolescents who've physically attacked parents in the past should be taken more seriously than threats from children who have never hurt anyone. Parents are often goaded into angry or violent reactions because of how frightening or threatening their children seem.

♦ Therapists tend to err in the direction of assessing greater danger with aggressive teenagers than the situation warrants. Therefore, they should look closely for evidence that a less ominous prognosis is appropriate. The fact that an adolescent didn't actually hit anyone with a brandished hammer is often obscured by everyone's fear over how close the adolescent came to actually hitting the person.

♦ Therapists are influenced by the feelings that parents communicate during sessions. Therapists who notice themselves having strong feelings of anger, fear, or hopelessness when dealing with adolescents must become knowledgeable about the origin of those feelings and more adept at recognizing when they are triggered, so that they can minimize their influence on the assessment. Therapists may be receiving those feelings from family members. For instance, a frightened parent may lead a therapist to feel more endangered than the situation warrants by using frightening and inflammatory language or tone of voice.

SOOTHING THE PETULANT CHILD:
INTERVENTION AT LEVEL 1

Adolescents at Level 1 act mildly dramatic under the assumption that at least one of their parents has a soft heart. If a teenager bats .500 at hitting a parent's soft heart—that is, if he or she manages to create doubt and guilt in one parent—the mission of keeping parents from agreeing has been accomplished. If both parents are devastated and guilt-ridden by their child's emotional outbursts, they will most likely stop any course of action that was designed to put pressure on the young person to change. Even in a single-parent family there's usually another adult involved, such as a grandparent, who functions as the other half of the parenting pair and is the other target.

One parent may react guiltily or sympathetically toward the exploding teenager, a reaction that either makes it more difficult for the other parent to stand firm or leads that parent into a more extreme posture to compensate for the mate's ambivalence. An adolescent who generates guilt or sympathy is usually in control of the family interaction because any attempt on the forceful parent's part to follow through with decisive action will be met with anger and criticism from the other parent. Once parents begin an angry struggle, any attempt by one parent to intervene with the child will peter out into nothingness. Anger between the parents then paralyzes them both, preventing further attempts at asserting parental power, and strengthens the adolescent's position in the family.

Straightforward behavior management techniques work effectively with aggression at Level 1—*if* both parents can be convinced to carry them out. For instance, simple reward procedures or logical consequences may be used. Much like a preschooler's temper tantrum, if the adolescent's protest falls on deaf ears and he or she doesn't succeed in getting the desired change, the behavior will often disappear after a series of such failed attempts. As with any plan to extinguish unwanted behavior, parents must understand that the troubled behavior will escalate before it goes away. It's human nature to try harder before giving up on a plan. If parents are told about this expected increase that precedes improvement, they're less likely to become discouraged when the momentary increase happens.

I recently learned of a charming example of a simple but effective reward procedure for young siblings whose arguments have become too frequent and intense. Each week the children are each given an age-appropriate set amount of money in change above and beyond their usual allowance, for instance, a roll of dimes. A coin is removed each time the children argue. The children get to keep whatever money they have left at the end of the week. This approach has the advantage of using both the carrot and the stick; reward and punishment are being used at once. This technique could also be used to intervene with children who talk back to their parents or display other aggressive responses (e.g., door slamming). The amount of money used would increase depending on the age of the children.

Although at some levels of aggressiveness young people respond well to humor, this sort of response doesn't seem to be too successful at this level. There's no harm in encouraging parents to respond with humor, but the young person at this stage may react like a grumpy 4-year-old who just woke up from a nap. If parents get a bad reaction, they must be ready and able to gracefully stop the attempt at humor and try something else.

Before attempting to be humorous, parents must be asked two questions:

1. Does their child have a sense of humor? That is, can the child laugh at him- or herself when not upset?
2. Can the parents be humorous in a playful, teasing manner without being cruel or sarcastic?

If the answer to each question is yes, they can proceed. An example of a humorous response might be for a parent to act melodramatically affectionate at a time when he or she would otherwise be reacting angrily or argumentatively. Gentle teasing may also be tried. Parents might respond to door slamming by encouraging the child to slam it again, noting that the last attempt was kind of feeble and not worthy of being called a slam. Again, such teasing has to be presented playfully rather than sarcastically if there's any hope of succeeding in defusing the situation. The point isn't so much for the parent to be clever or tricky but simply to do something to avoid playing out the usual cycle of control and rebellion.

Attempts by parents to reason with an adolescent at Level 1 may get the same response as an attempt to reason with a 4-year-old who's having a tantrum. However, before most parents will agree to ignore or otherwise extinguish their child's behavior, they usually have to try to reason with the child first. Parents may need to be coached in a specific way of speaking to their child in an attempt to have a reasonable interaction. The therapist can help parents give specific instructions to their child to stop a particular behavior so that there can be a discussion. Parents can then have a conversation with the child about the negative behavior and about how his or her point could be made without resorting to behaviors that can't be allowed.

Adolescents are impulsive and often don't have a clear understanding of future gratification. They become caught up in the need they feel at the time. If they can be helped to see a greater benefit in the future as a result of controlling impulsive behavior in the present, they've learned a valuable lesson about, as my grandmother would say, not cutting off your nose to spite your face.

If attempts by parents to reason with their child fail, the therapist should begin helping parents use extinction techniques. If parents keep trying to talk at an upset teenager they can escalate the situation into one that produces Level 2 behavior from the child. Extinction can best be achieved by ignoring unwanted behavior as completely as possible. When parents refuse to respond to an outburst, the teenager finds it disorienting. When their behavior is being ignored, adolescents who have angrily demanded to be left alone may even seek out their parents a short time later to find out what's going on. When this happens, it should be understood as a sign of parents regaining control of their family.

I've often directed parents to act affectionately toward each other in place of responding to the child. For example, a husband might be told to kiss his wife on the lips whenever their son begins whining at her. If the boy continues, the husband should kiss her again. While kissing each other, parents aren't giving a response to their son and both feel more unified as a couple. It's also hard for the mother to give any response to the child, including reversing her decision, when her lips are occupied. A mother can also be directed to kiss her husband instead of responding to a whining child. Parents have only refused this directive when the marriage was so bad that there was nothing but hatred left between them. If parents refuse the kissing strategy, the therapist learns that the marriage is the greater problem and can then deal with the marital conflict directly.

Confusion Techniques

Confusion techniques can be powerful at Level 1. These techniques involve a change in parental response that a young person will find disorienting. Human beings are creatures of habit. We tend to do things the same way over time and expect predictable responses from others. How many of us put our clothes on in a different order each morning or wash body parts in the shower in random order? Because others are also human, they usually don't let us down; that is, they give the anticipated response. Most arguments with parents happen when the adolescent already anticipates what the parents will say and do; the teenager has already decided on his or her next response or action before the parents even speak. When parents respond in ways that aren't anticipated young people begin to hesitate, which causes them to momentarily lose their usual confidence. Parents may even see evidence of this state of confusion as the teenager slips briefly into a trance to reorganize and figure out how to respond.

Consider, for example, 11-year-old Mary, who became enraged when her mother asked her to clean her room when she preferred going to her friend's house. At first Mary sulked to see whether she could elicit enough sympathy and anxiety to get her mother to give in to her desire to go to her friend's house. When her mother held her ground, Mary became angry and began to exhibit the first stages of a tantrum during which she always said things like, "This isn't fair" or "This is ridiculous." At this point it was possible for Mary's mother to use a confusion-based response rather than withdraw from the struggle to avoid conflict and hurt between herself and her daughter. Under ordinary circumstances Mary's mother would see her daughter's pain and give in to her demands. The few times she stuck to her guns, Mary's mother felt so bad because her daughter was angry at her that she apologized to Mary after successfully getting her to do as she was told. A shift was possible in the struggle between Mary and her mother that wouldn't require the mother to relent in the usual way. Such a change could also reduce the likelihood that the situation would progress to a Level 2 problem because of a mutual escalation of anger in parent and child.

What would happen if Mary's mother were to respond to the beginning of Mary's tantrum by immediately giving her daughter a hug and a kiss and telling her how much she loved her? Would-be behaviorists would gasp at this suggestion and claim that a hug and kiss would reward the escalation. However, the power of this new maternal response to confuse the existing sequence of interactions is much greater than any possible simple reinforcement. Parents are often astonished by how paralyzed their children become as they try to make some sense of an unexpected parental response. Parents then witness a change in their children's predictable behaviors. The therapist can use this opening to facilitate a healthy conversation, a negotiation, or some other positive change. The disorientation adolescents experience at this time leaves them temporarily suggestible, so they tend to go along with whatever new direction the therapist begins. Again, the point is to avoid playing into the usual cycle of control and rebellion.

It may be necessary to convince parents that an affectionate response is in order. Parents often ask, "How can I do that when I don't feel like it?" In Mary's case the therapist pointed out to her mother all the losses and unhappy circumstances that had occurred in Mary's life and was able to redefine her behavior as an attempt to keep her parents close and emotionally involved with her for security's sake. People can't be much closer than when they're nose to nose and angry at each other.

Reversing the Balance of Power

In order to upset ritualized responses, it may be useful to reverse the balance of power. When there are disagreements between parents that result in Level 1 aggression, there's usually one parent who considers himself or herself the expert on discipline—despite both parents' dismal level of success. The parent who has mishandled discipline in the past typically withdraws from parenting, which increases the isolation and anger the disciplining parent feels. The parental cycle of anger and withdrawal gets worse and worse until the child erupts. A parent may have been alcoholic or drug addicted and unavailable. He or she may have always put work or family of origin before the children and spouse. A serious depression might have sent a parent into retreat for months or years.

Commonly (but not always), the withdrawn parent is the father and the overinvolved parent the mother. No matter which parent is peripheral (i.e., less involved), the therapist should look for signs that both spouses are open to reestablishing a cooperative relationship as parents. Signs that show hope for successfully rebuilding the parental team are the following:

♦ Does the overinvolved parent say that the distant parent is welcome to be more active? That is, does he or she invite the other back into the fold?

♦ If not, does the overinvolved parent still scold the peripheral parent for not being sufficiently involved? This way of asking the distant spouse for help allows the therapist to discuss ways that the peripheral parent can become involved, regardless of how reluctant the more central parent may be.

♦ Does the peripheral parent express willingness to be involved?

♦ If there have been seriously inappropriate behaviors by the peripheral parent (i.e., violence, drunkenness, or abandoning the family), does he or she understand these to be inappropriate and show a willingness to do better?

♦ Do the children, when spoken to alone, express some affection or desire for the peripheral parent? Or are they at least equally negative about both their parents?

If these questions are met with encouraging responses, the therapist can proceed. The parents can be asked to make the offending youngster answerable completely to the peripheral parent for a week. Who can handle the child best isn't important when using this technique, once danger has been properly assessed; what's important is the way this tactic forces the teenager to totally rethink his or her ritualized responses. Those responses are usually organized around planning countermaneuvers to the attempts at discipline that come from the more overinvolved parent. This approach causes confusion in the teenager when the usual foe stops being reactive and says, "Wait until your father (or mother) gets home."

When parents aren't yet ready to cooperate with each other the therapist can use a slight modification of the strategy just described. Either parent can be put in charge of correcting the child for a week. When that parent fails, the other is then put in charge for a week. When both have failed to change their child's behavior, the therapist can conclude that neither can do it alone and that teamwork is necessary.

This reversing of the balance involves simple reformulations of the usual and expected response patterns by parents, siblings, and other significant family members. School personnel can also be coached to change expected responses to disrupt a student's ritualized reactions. Similar strategies can be devised for any other professionals involved.

At Level 1 the problem doesn't have to be approached as an adversarial situation. In many cases a discussion with the parents and child separately provides enough information to identify a simple solution. An entire problem might begin with a teenager who's angry because he or she thinks a curfew is unfair. That is, a simple grievance may underlie Level 1 or 2 aggression. Power hasn't become a major tool of interaction yet, and the young person will often give up the aggressive approach to solving problems if the issues involved can be discussed and resolved. Resolution usually isn't accomplished through expression of feelings but by identifying and solving the problems the aggressive behavior is trying to influence.

A FLAIR FOR THE DRAMATIC: INTERVENTION AT LEVEL 2

Level 2 is distinguished from Level 1 by the escalation of anger and the beginning of a verbal assault. It's likely that one or both parents will respond angrily to an adolescent when confronted directly. Therapists will notice the growing ability of the teenager at Level 2 to incapacitate the parents by using aggression to enrage them. At Level 1 children engender sympathy and may get their way. At Level 2 children see that they can inflame their parents to the point where the parents' emotions take charge of their good sense. If one parent becomes verbally aggressive, the potential for an incapacitating conflict between the parents increases dramatically. Disagreement between the parents can become intense enough to continue beyond the struggle with their child and may interfere with their marriage.

This new level of aggression may be a simple behavioral escalation, but it may also point out the beginning of emotional concerns in the family that aren't getting resolved and are upsetting the children. A marital conflict that's beginning to look damaging can cause a child to act enraged, thus drawing the issue of anger out in the open so it can be addressed. For example, a daughter may engage in a verbal struggle with her father that looks just like the father's arguments with her mother. When he argues with his daughter about how poor her choice of friends is, the father may be expressing his anger over his wife's having male friends. Because the issue of appropriate friends is now raised regularly by their daughter and can be discussed through her, the parents stop arguing the way they once did (Madanes, 1984). The tendency in such a metaphorical argument would be for the mother to defend her daughter and argue that she should be trusted and allowed to choose her own friends.

Level 2 aggression may occur when a parent has become depressed or isn't recovering from the death of a loved one. If a depressed parent can be provoked to rage, he or she pulls out of the depression for a while, having expressed the underlying rage. It's better, though, if the therapist doesn't become overly analytical at this point. The same interventions that were effective at Level 1 may also disrupt the development of further behavioral problems at this level of aggression; that is, behavioral and confusion techniques are often sufficient to correct the adolescent mis-behavior. The presence of depression or other emotional problems in the parent may never become an issue, or the troubled parent may ask for help as the child's problem improves.

The degree of difficulty in getting parents to use extinction tech-niques goes up a bit when the adolescent's aggression is at Level 2. Parents are witnessing the rage of children who are beginning to call them names and blame them for every perceived injustice. Children punishing their parents by withdrawing love and approval is a serious attack that increases the level of paralysis experienced by parents.

If a parent who is usually able to deal with a child's behavior becomes paralyzed by the child's withdrawal of love, the therapist should try to increase the parent's resolve to stick to his or her position. Increasing parental resolve is often accomplished by getting another adult to team up with the parent. A peripheral parent may be encouraged to get involved when there are two parents in the home, and a single parent may wind up using an aunt, uncle, or grandparent to increase the power of the parental unit. Divorced parents can be brought together to act as a team if they have a cooperative relationship. If conflict between divorced parents is contributing to the problem, the therapist may need to see them without the child to resolve differences and begin a new spirit of cooperation. At Level 2 there's a question as to whether the individual resolve of one parental figure will be sufficient to overcome the verbal assaults of an adolescent. Forming a coalition with another adult often gives parents more structure within which to stick to their resolve because they've agreed on a course of action with a teammate. When such a coalition exists, a young person is more likely to believe that a promised consequence will occur and may decide not to misbehave.

Electing a Godparent

Cloé Madanes has begun asking single parents to elect godparents for their children. A well-chosen godparent can be not only a good adult influence on the child but a partner for the parent. A common response from isolated single parents is that no one exists who could help them manage a difficult teenager. Encouragement by the therapist to discuss godparenthood with relatives and friends often results in finding a helper who's flattered at having been chosen as a person with special qualities. An isolated single mother may be encouraged to ask her brother to build a special relationship with his nephew. The uncle would be a wise choice if the nephew has always respected him or if the uncle has the strength of character that the situation requires. While spending time with his nephew at sporting events or in other recreational activities, an uncle could initiate a discussion about appropriate male behavior and take a strong position. At higher levels of aggression he can be called on to deal with physical threats, if necessary.

Isolated people may come to rely too heavily on helping profession-als. When dependent parents are asked who would be a good godparent, they may immediately choose the school counselor or a social services worker. It's best to discourage a parent from selecting such a professional for the godparent role because that person's presence is temporary. Moreover, professionals can't be asked to do many of the things a friend or relative might be willing to do—for example, being on 24-hour call for emergencies or physically restraining a teenager. Furthermore, a discouraged parent would be tempted to take a back seat to a godparent who's a professional and would wait for the expert to take action whereas he or she might be more likely to take charge with the assistance of a friend or relative.

The Pawnbroker

From Level 2 through Level 4 the pawnbroker technique offers a way of increasing consequences that may prevent an adolescent's aggressive acting out from reaching higher levels. Parents may have already tried a variety of punishments and consequences only to find that their adoles-cent has either become insensitive to them or found ways around them. In the pawnbroker technique the parents are asked to identify behavior that goes beyond what's acceptable. Usually these serious infractions include violence, disrespect toward parents or other adults, threats (direct or implied), and a variety of forms of verbal abusiveness. The therapist asks parents to cut pieces of paper into one hundred small slips to serve as tickets, each with a specific fine attached to it. For instance, each ticket given could cost the adolescent one dollar. The amount of the fine is best determined by what would constitute a painful consequence for misbehavior, but a parent should allow the young person some opportunity to learn from experience prior to exhausting his or her funds. A ticket is issued each time the child behaves in one of the identified unacceptable ways. It's best for a parent to design a ticket that can be torn in half so that both parent and child can have evidence that a ticket has been issued; the first tickets issued often find their way into the wastebasket.

The therapist can explain to parents that their teenager isn't sufficiently aware of the disrespect involved in certain ways of acting and must therefore be sensitized to how others are reacting to certain behaviors; Children and teenagers who act out aggressively are often undersocialized; they are often more ignorant than evil. They're at a stage where they're too focused on themselves to be aware of their effect on others. Parents who have overindulged their children's feelings are more likely to take a powerful step if that step is in the interest of teaching rather than punishment. The pawnbroker approach has an educational element that adds a bit of sugar to the medicine for kindly parents.

Teenagers who are deprived of their allowance as a form of discipline will inevitably point out that they don't have any money to pay a fine. To deal with this maneuver, children may be allowed to settle their debt through services. If they are unwilling to work off the debt, their parents can begin to repossess belongings. The repossession could involve, for example, one cassette or compact disk at a time. Stereo equipment, designer clothes, and video games are usually powerful targets. One stereo speaker is a small item whose absence can make a large impact on a teenager. Nevertheless, teenagers who are presented with the pawnbroker technique will usually declare that they don't care what the parents take; this is either because they don't believe their parents will actually take anything or because they've always been able to get things back that were taken. The power of the pawnbroker technique is that each possession taken is to be considered pawned with the parents and must be bought back with money or services within 30 days. The adolescent is given a pawn ticket or receipt. At the end of 30 days, the pawned possessions are sold or given to charity. To help parents accept losing things they paid for, the donation can be taken as a tax deduction. If the therapist's explanations aren't enough to convince parents to be tough, he or she can point out that playing pawnbroker is cheaper than long-term therapy or hospitalization.

Adolescents typically complain that the pawned possessions are theirs and that their parents have no right to take them. The therapist can explain that possessions in life are often sold to pay debts. This reasonable explanation is usually sufficient to reduce the parents' guilt and increase their resolve; in addition, the therapist can remind the parents that the pawnbroker technique is being done for the educational benefit of the young person, not as a punishment. Teenagers may also say it's okay for their parents to take things because the parents paid for them in the first place and they're only punishing themselves. The therapist can point out that the pawning of possessions won't cost the parents anything because they won't need to replace the repossessed items once they're given away.

Level 2 is still a stage at which there need not be an assumption of significant disturbance. As with Level 1, straightforward discussion, negotiation, and deal making may resolve the entire issue. These adolescents haven't controlled adults with aggression long enough to be hooked on this way of solving problems.

WHAT TO DO WHEN DAMAGE BEGINS: INTERVENTION AT LEVEL 3

Real fear begins in the hearts of parents when their adolescent's aggression is at Level 3. Their child has now moved from indirect threats and verbal aggression to overt verbal threats of injury to parents, siblings, and pets and minor damage to possessions. Until Level 3 is reached, parents can continue to believe in the benevolence of their children. Now parents must begin to question whether their children are truly hateful and even dangerous to the people who love them. The entire family becomes focused on whether aggression will continue into Levels 4 and above or be stopped at this stage.

Humor and confusion techniques that failed at Level 2 will, in all likelihood, fail if aggression continues to Level 3. If humor and confusion techniques were going to be effective with a particular child, they would have interrupted the development of his or her abusiveness at Level 2, and Level 3 would never have been reached. If, however, the parents or caretakers (as in a group home or foster home) didn't attempt humor- or confusion-based alternatives at Level 2, it's reasonable to attempt them now. For example, parents might respond to a threat as if they believe their son or daughter is joking; sometimes an adolescent will allow the situation to be detoxified by accepting the parents' playfulness and withdrawing the threat. It should be noted, though, that if attempts at humor and confusion don't succeed fairly rapidly (i.e., after 1 or 2 weeks of consistently attempting to respond in these new ways), they should be abandoned. Continuation of a failing approach costs the parental team a great deal of power and credibility, which they can't afford to lose.

At Level 3 the therapist's understanding of an adolescent's motivation may need to move from an assumption of benevolence to a belief that the adolescent is wielding power. What could previously be accomplished with humor, negotiation, or confusion now requires skill in the art of power brokering. Parents must be willing to see their children as malicious or, at the very least, as out of control.

To avoid being victimized by powerful threats, parents must put aside their benevolence to some extent. They must begin to realize they're in a contest where they must, in order to ensure their children's future, exert parental authority and organize deliberate, powerful strategies for blocking their children's growing escalations. Therapists must help turn parents' fear into a new resolve to take charge of the situation and must encourage a strong belief in their ability to do so.

Even at this moderate level of aggression, parents may be tired and worn down. Disappointment over family struggles and years of guilt may have left parents depressed. Tirades and threats of retaliation gradually wear on parents, leaving them paralyzed by fear. When a daughter who played with fire as a child threatens to burn the house down while her parents are sleeping, parents may develop a stronger and stronger belief that she really might do so. Words alone can be very powerful. As parents become more worn out and discouraged, their fears become greater, leaving them with even less energy to take action. Parents may even believe their child could resort to some extreme act, such as burning the house down, without ever making the threat.

At Level 3 adolescents usually won't hurt themselves directly. However, they pay close attention to finding ways of upsetting others without endangering themselves. The greater danger is that parents will try to establish their authority by use of psychiatric intervention and thereby lose what little power they still have. A lot of the teenagers brought to therapy by their parents have been in previous therapy where they were seen individually. Parents were kept in the dark as to the content of the therapy or the status of their children's mental health. This affront to parental authority by therapists, and the fact that parents allowed the secrecy, cost them what little respect they had in the eyes of their children. In conjoint sessions or parental consultation sessions parents may even be blamed by therapists for their inequities in raising and handling their children.

Once again, the critical step in therapy is to establish the parents as authorities and make it clear to children that they have little direct power over the situation but will be listened to respectfully. A generational boundary must be established that distinguishes between levels of family hierarchy and clarifies the power each level possesses (Minuchin, 1974). Most aggressive teenagers act as if there's no difference in authority between adults and children and speak as if they are their parents' equals. Absence of generational boundaries is dramatized by the common adolescent statement "I won't act respectfully toward them [their parents] until they act respectfully toward me."

The therapist's first job is to reestablish the parents as the experts on their child and to present him- or herself as a consultant who works for them. Parents set the goals for change. The therapist begins assessing the parents' level of competence and power in the first session, with the goal of helping them develop the clout necessary to take charge of their child's life. The process of helping parents regain their authority presents a dilemma in itself. If a therapist tells parents they should be in better control of their child, that therapist is actually declaring his or her own control by criticizing the parents. The parents, in turn, might then assume that the therapist should be in charge and might respond by relegating their authority to the therapist. Therapists can create an atmosphere conducive to reestablishing parental authority by first listening closely to the parents and asking them for more detail. Therapists often make the mistake of moving to a teaching posture very early in therapy; their lecturing tells parents that they don't have what it takes to solve their own problems. Even questionable attitudes by parents are best not challenged at this point.

Right from the beginning a therapist should tell parents that no one can solve their child's problem but them. If previous therapy for the problem has failed, the therapist can emphasize that the professionals haven't succeeded. Otherwise the parents wouldn't be sitting in the therapist's office. Parents should be encouraged to believe that the wisdom necessary to help their child is within them just waiting to come out. Another way for the therapist to challenge the parents without preaching is to wonder out loud why they haven't taken charge up to this point. If the therapist voices the assumption that there's a good reason why they haven't assumed control, the parents will typically begin to discuss these reasons. Once it's clear that they won't be blamed, parents feel free to take charge. Even directives can be given in a way that avoids taking control away from the parents. To offer the parents strategies without entering the realm of teaching and preaching, the therapist can say something like, "Here's an idea you might not have tried. How about giving it a try for a week?"

Parents must be helped to understand that the platitudes their children throw at them about trust, fairness, and being from the Dark Ages need not be responded to with parental guilt. Moralistic statements may be discussed by applying the issue of fairness to parents also. Parents may say, "I've tried to be fair with you, but now I think it's only fair for you to at least listen to my view of the situation." Parents can offer to later discuss the fairness of a decision on which they expect immediate compliance by saying, "We can discuss the fairness of our decision at 3 o'clock when you come home from school tomorrow. If we agree with your point of view, we won't ask you to do this again." Detouring the discussion changes the issue away from a struggle over who's going to win.

Power is the immediate issue at Level 3; benevolence has failed. Therefore, parents must be encouraged to react calmly and deliberately to their children's threats and discouraged from threatening their children in return or lamely lecturing them. Obviously, therapists themselves must avoid lecturing as they guide parents toward better relations with their children. An example of the distinction between meaningless threats and calm but firm action is the difference between telling a teenager for the fifth time that he won't be allowed to go to the prom, and tearing up the prom tickets in front of him. Parents often make threats they can't carry out and then lose power when their children call their bluff. More importantly, as parents argue with their children, everyone becomes increasingly upset. Emotional upset leads both parents and children to say things they don't mean and can escalate an adolescent's aggression from Level 2 to Level 3 or 4.

The task for therapists is learning how to tell parents to stop criticizing, threatening, and lecturing without undermining their authority by criticizing their techniques. If the therapist lectures, the parents will go home and lecture their child. If the therapist scolds, the parents will go home and scold their child. A gentler method is to ask parents to list each of the methods they've used to intervene with their child's behavior and then discuss which ones have worked and which ones have failed. Once their previous methods have been divided into successes and failures, parents will usually agree that they should stop fruitless tactics. Parents can be asked, "Which of these approaches would you like to keep and which should we replace with something new?"

Arguments with their children can be avoided if parents understand that the rule about giving children fair warning of consequences isn't valid when adolescents get out of control. Once power tactics are being used by teenagers they give up the right to hear an explanation for their parents' decisions and plans.

Adolescents begin to conceal more and more information about where they're going, what they're doing, or what they're thinking. Parents often say they don't feel they know their child the way they once did. The adolescent who displays Level 3 aggression is in a transitional stage where the struggle for power hasn't taken on pathological proportions yet and the young person's level of secrecy hasn't become extreme. Parents can regain a great deal of power and control by actively seeking out information they've hesitated to obtain in the past. Parents should be encouraged to meet with all teachers and school administrators involved with their child. They have a right to know where their children are and who their friends are, as well as what the friends are like and who their parents are. Despite a teenager's heart-rending attacks of "You're checking up on me!" what's learned by getting information provides parents with ideas about how to regain power and get back in control of the situation. This process of information gathering may lead to the discovery that a child is involved with alcohol and drugs, gangs, or just plain bad company, any of which can encourage irresponsibility and disrespect.

One obvious advantage to parents' learning more about their children's activities is the development of a network of concerned adults who share information, something the adolescents have been doing with each other for years. Parents can form coalitions to bring the children of two or three families under control through one set of actions coordinated by a therapist. Imagine the impact if several sets of parents showed up together at an unsupervised party their children had gone to without permission. As parents form coalitions and gain information, they become progressively more powerful and, consequently, more motivated.

THREATENING GESTURES AND SERIOUS DAMAGE TO POSSESSIONS: INTERVENTION AT LEVEL 4

When a child's aggression reaches Level 4, the intensity of the threats being made increase dramatically. These adolescents consistently make aggressive responses to any unpopular position their parents take and then act this anger out against objects. Although many normal teenagers put an occasional hole in a wall or door, adolescents with Level 4 aggression do damage consistently. Their aggressive acts are often targeted directly at parents and their possessions, in contrast to normal kids who go to their room when enraged and break their own things. Adolescents who damage their parents' possessions have crossed the generational boundary and are acting as if they have the right to punish their parents.

Here's an example of a case of Level 4 aggression: A 14-year-old boy's single mother took away his CD player because he skipped school. He retaliated by smashing her clock radio on the floor. When his mother grounded him for breaking her radio, the boy grabbed the curtains she was hanging and ripped them off the wall. The boy then picked up the hammer his mother had been using and threatened to kill her with it.

Surprisingly, when therapists speak to such adolescents one-on-one, some of them (albeit a small percentage) are willing to discuss their concerns about their family, school, or friends. Therefore, a therapist should always try to have a private talk with an adolescent before assuming there's going to be a struggle. Everyone's life is simplified if adolescents discuss the problems they want to solve. If they share their concerns with a therapist, they may agree to stop all aggression in exchange for the therapist's agreeing to influence their parents or teachers on reasonable issues. Knowledge of this coalition between therapist and adolescent is best kept between the two of them. Such a coalition should only be made if the adolescent seems sincere; otherwise, he or she could easily go to the parents and repeat things the therapist said privately in an out-of-context, incriminating way. Although negotiating and making a deal with an adolescent is desirable and should be tried, it's best for the therapist to remember that power is now in primary play, and the contest will often have to be held on a battleground rather than at the negotiating table. If a therapist is uncertain of a teenager's sincerity, it's a gamble to make a deal. If the teenager doesn't keep the initial agreement, parents may see the therapist as a gullible do-gooder who got taken in, and they may drop out of therapy. On the other hand, if the therapist gambles and the teenager cooperates, the entire therapy will be much less painful for everyone.

In situations where parents aren't physically (or emotionally) able to protect themselves, it's crucial that protectors be found. Often a male relative or neighbor can be found whose presence inspires respect in the teenager. Protectors should be invited to therapy sessions. They can remain on call if dangerous situations occur. In one such situation the parent gave a beeper to the support person to ensure her ability to get help quickly. Such a coalition between adults is very effective in convincing adolescents that they have to find other ways of getting what they want. (A 13-year-old boy told me in his first therapy session that the problem was simply that he wanted his way and wouldn't take no for an answer.)

It's usually best to view aggression as the behavior of adolescents who want their way, whether they admit to being stubborn or not. Some children say that they don't know what comes over them, that they just lose control of themselves. Young people who claim their behavior happens outside their awareness are particularly troublesome because such a response is a perfect opening for the institution of intensive psychiatric care. Parents who believe their child is mad rather than bad are more likely to tolerate aggressive behavior and to seek a psychiatric expert who will "fix" the child. However, handing a child over to a professional reduces the power of the parents and thereby increases the danger of further aggression from the child.

Unfortunately, in some situations there simply isn't anyone who can be found to be a protective support person for a beleaguered parent. If legal authorities must become involved, it's better that they get involved at the request of parents. A therapist can help parents learn to use the legal system efficiently and can guide them through the steps. As is true with earlier levels of adolescent aggression, hospitals and individual therapists are best avoided because their involvement implies a mental illness that moves the case out of the parents' domain. Parents may take steps to deal with misbehavior, but it's unlikely they'll feel confident taking steps to correct a child who has been diagnosed with, for instance, bipolar disorder.

Therapists must come to terms with how they conceptualize the problem of adolescent aggression. If aggression is seen as the result of mental illness or psychopathology, it follows that aggressive behavior is involuntary and out of the teenager's control. On the other hand, if aggressive acts are seen as misbehavior, then it follows that the aggression is voluntary and is therefore a behavior the adolescent can choose to stop. It is also true that if aggressive behavior is viewed as being out of the adolescent's control, parents can't insist that their child stop acting that way and have no authority to bring about change. However, if their teenager is understood to be misbehaving, parents are clearly the experts, because correction of behavior problems is a parent's job; simply put, the behavior isn't being excused by professional experts.

If a therapist decides that other professionals are necessary, the criminal justice system is usually a more helpful first step than a psychiatric hospital. The attribution of criminal intent continues to define adolescent aggression as voluntary, intentional, and punishable. Most psychiatric hospitals are fairly pleasant for adolescents and only punish parents—when they get the bill for the amount their insurance didn't cover. Any improvement in a teenager's reliance on violent behavior after a psychiatric hospitalization is typically short-lived once he or she is back home dealing with all the same people and situations. Hospitals are indicated when family members can't be organized to provide safety, the courts and police can't or won't act, and people are in imminent danger.

Whether or not to recommend that parents use the police in dealing with their child should be decided only after the therapist has acquired knowledge about and experience with the police force in a given locality. In some towns police never show up on a domestic violence call; in other towns, they respond rapidly and forcefully. In the example in Chapter 5 of the 14-year-old boy who threatened his mother with a hammer, the therapist knew that the police in that city responded well—and even bent the rules a bit—in attempting to frighten teens away from a life of crime. When the boy threatened his mother, she called the police, and, as expected, an officer the size of a linebacker showed up in 15 minutes. As you may recall, the officer attempted to reason with the boy and was promptly told by the teen, "Fuck you, pig!" Issuing this statement turned out to be a serious misjudgment on the young man's part. Although the officer didn't hurt the boy, he handled him in a manner that left little doubt that he could.

The officer left a pale young man in his mother's care. This case remained in therapy for two more sessions, with no further incidents, and then terminated. The boy's grades improved, and he stopped threatening his mother. Follow-up at 1 year found him still doing pretty well and behaving toward his mother in a relatively courteous manner. There had been no further bouts of abnormal aggression, and he continued to go to school and do adequately. This case ended happily, but police authorities shouldn't be called if a town's police force is known for inaction in cases of domestic violence involving an adolescent. If a parent contacts the police and authorities do little or nothing, the chances increase of that parent being further victimized. Therapists can avoid the error of recommending police intervention in communities where this tactic would be ineffective by meeting the youth officers in their clients' communities first and knowing them by name.

A range of power tactics may be used by parents whose children's aggression is at Level 4. At the very least, parents must be prepared to use much stronger consequences than they typically would. When problems are moderately severe, parents must discover where they truly have power they can barter with. These areas of power can be identified by asking parents to describe the range of services they currently provide for their children. Therapists can then help parents see that they can exercise control, if they so choose, by reducing these services (e.g., financial support, transportation, and meal preparation).

Young people who are acting up usually aren't doing much to help around the house. Parents report that since it's so hard to get their adolescent to do anything, it's easier for them to do the work themselves. Teenagers may not avoid household duties at earlier levels of aggression but can be counted on to do little or nothing at Level 4. Moreover, parents of these teens often don't know where their children are when they leave the house or when they'll be back. The teenagers may be skipping school; even if they attend classes, they may not be doing class assignments and homework—although some teenagers act out by doing homework and never turning it in. If the adolescent is demonstrating problems only with chores and school, parents should respond as if it's a Level 3 situation. Level 3 interventions will either correct the situation or escalate it to where the symptoms clearly define the behavior as Level 4.

Parents cook meals, provide money, and allow liberal use of the family car. They're often so thrilled when their child allows them to help that they do so gratefully. Helping their child is the only reassurance many parents have that they're still in the child's life. For example, parents drive their kids to the mall or to sports events and gladly replace broken sports equipment, feeling it unfair to deprive a troubled teenager of a healthy outlet like a favorite sport. They may also feel coerced into providing transportation because of their fear that someone they've never met will be driving or that their children will hitchhike.

Because most parents provide their children with funds and help them in a variety of ways, changing the amount or types of assistance they give is a powerful way parents can intervene. Removing various services in response to being mistreated by their children can demonstrate that parents mean business and won't give endlessly. Therapists can encourage parents to handle the problem playfully yet powerfully by going right out and buying supplies to make signs with slogans such as PARENTS ON STRIKE AGAINST UNGRATEFUL CHILDREN (see "Angry at the World" in Chapter 5). Parents can picket the front of the house during their free time (when they'd otherwise be providing services) and can stop all financial outlay as part of the strike. Then, as with any strike, the parents wait the adolescent out; they can encourage the child to present written demands that can be addressed in negotiations. As with previous levels of adolescent aggression, a coalition with an outside adult may be required to provide enough momentum when a parent's resolve is inadequate to carry through with the consequences of a stand that has been taken. The idea of a strike may seem extreme, but it has a humorous quality to it. This is best done with older adolescents or young adults to avoid charges of parental neglect. If their child is 15 or 16, parents can bring groceries home but can stop cooking; they can also cease buying anything the child really likes.

The idea of a strike was inspired by the actions taken by the city of Key West, Florida. In the late 1970s a customs checkpoint was established between Key West and the mainland to reduce drug trafficking. Tourism was harmed. When the government refused to remove the customs checkpoint, the mayor of Key West publicly announced that Key West was seceding from the union. The people of Key West would no longer be Americans and would in the future be called Conchs. The island of Key West would be called the Conch Republic. Obviously, this meant that Key West residents would no longer pay taxes to the U.S. government. Key West's argument was sound: If they were to be treated as a foreign country, they would become one. Within a few weeks the customs checkpoint was removed. Humorous solutions can be powerful.

In another instance, a strike was carried out by a widowed father of three girls, ages 15, 16, and 17. The girls would team up and harass him unmercifully about what a bad father he had always been. No matter how attentive he became, they would never forgive him. They swore at him and left him in tears. The abuse resulted in the father feeling so hurt and guilty that he never stopped his daughters from doing anything they wanted, which reinforced their perception that he didn't care. He finally decided something had to be done, so he went on strike as a show of force. The strike was particularly appropriate because the girls' father had been doing all the housework and the strike forced his daughters to do more. As with people in Key West, the father reasoned that as long as he was being treated in a certain way, he might as well begin to act the part to make a point. The father didn't spend all of his free time picketing, but it was a great strategy for calming himself when he began to get fueled up for a verbal struggle with one of the girls. At the family's next therapy session, all three girls talked more freely about what needed to be changed at home, and their dad was able to go back on the job.

This idea of a strike might stimulate the reader to come up with additional ideas for interventions involving the services parents provide for their children. For example, Mary was a single mom who recently decided to take away the car she'd given her 16-year-old verbally abusive daughter, Renee. Mary had continued to pay for car insurance, repairs, and gasoline despite the way her daughter treated her. Mary had hesitated to take the car away because Renee helped take her 13-year-old sister places, which in turn helped Mary by relieving her of this chore. Mary finally decided to tie together the two issues—Renee's mistreatment of her and car use—and parked the car in a friend's garage until Renee followed her directions and spoke to her reasonably. Renee got the car back 5 weeks later, after making a lot of improvements in her attitude.

Level 4 is the first level where the "secret weapon strategy"—becomes appropriate. (The strategy is described fully in Chapter 8.) In the most serious of cases, families can consider sending a young person off to live with a friend or relative for a fixed length of time. They should be sent as far away as possible and to a place as unpleasant as possible. Jay Haley has recommended that parents move a person into their house to live for a period of time; the presence of an outsider often disrupts the spontaneity of ritualized aggressive escalations between parents and child.

TAKING ACTION WHEN PEOPLE GET HURT: INTERVENTION AT LEVEL 5

At Level 5, the struggle for power and control begins to take over and benevolence erodes. Family life is now dominated by conflict, and violence becomes physical. Although the origin of the symptom may be found in family problems, the atmosphere of violence, control, and struggle for power over others may be taking on a life of its own. Therefore, it is more important to focus on intervening in the violent cycle itself than to worry about why the symptom exists.

As with alcohol and drug addiction, aggression and violence require an assessment of whether or not the behavior is sufficiently self-reinforcing to be a problem in itself. If discussion of and feelings around an adolescent's aggression overshadow any attempt to discuss other family problems, it's best to view the aggression or violence as a problem in itself and start there. Intervention should focus on strategies for stopping the violence. The feelings behind and reasons for the violence are best set aside until the situation is safe. When their adolescent's aggression is stuck at this level, parents often continue to obsess about why their child would turn to such behavior; such parents don't believe any effective action can be taken until the underlying causes of the child's aggression are thoroughly understood. As described in Chapter 5, getting parents beyond this concern for underlying causes and motivating them to take action is a large part of the therapist's task.

With milder cases of Level 5 aggression, the following strategies may still be effective: confusion techniques, benevolent coalitions with the adolescent to help solve the family problems, and the pawn broker technique. As the level of true violence and risk increases, so does the need for parents to take control over what will be allowed to happen in the family. Greater violence requires greater use of interventions like the secret weapon strategy (see Chapter 8) or sending the young person to live with a friend or relative who won't be intimidated by aggressive behavior (strategies done at home should always be attempted first, before sending a young person away).

Techniques must focus on shifting the balance of power and putting authority back in the hands of parents (or other responsible adults). Coordination between all the adults involved is crucial; they must agree that the adolescent won't be told the content or outcome of adult meetings.

Parents may need to use physical management techniques to restrain a teenager and show him or her that violence won't be tolerated. The earlier physical restraint is used in cases of Level 5 aggression, the more likely it is to succeed. Restraint usually triggers an initial burst of counteraggression in the adolescent but is followed by submission if it's clear the adult doing the restraining won't relent in the face of threats. It's critical that restraint be done by those who aren't angry at the child and won't misuse the opportunity to act out their own anger in injurious ways. There are a variety of reasons why parents hesitate to physically restrain their children. Some simply feel it's wrong to use physical force with a child. Others fear further retaliation. Still others are afraid they'll be condemned by social agencies and taken to court as abusive parents.

It's a frightening thought for any parent to be in a physical struggle with one of their children. Yet, if adolescents don't learn that they'll be stopped from harming others by a family member, they might learn this lesson from the police or from someone on the street with a knife. Getting physical is risky and is only recommended when no other choices are available. If a teenager is closing in on a parent with a baseball bat in his hand, it's best for the parent to know how to stop him if he or she is cornered. Parents might seek out a physical management course like those given to social services and hospital personnel. Such courses teach how to restrain and incapacitate a violent person without doing harm.

With young adults and older teenagers a step can be taken toward restoring parental authority by using a technique developed by Mara Selvini Palazzoli (Palazzoli, Cirillo, Selvini, & Sorrentino, 1989). Although the technique has been discredited as an invariant prescription for use in all cases, the approach has merit in some situations when parents are trying to set proper boundaries. Palazzoli's prescription helps pull the parental couple into a secret coalition while encouraging them to begin looking at themselves as a couple who might have a life together. In this approach the parents leave a note for their kids that says they've gone out; then they simply disappear for at least a day and a night. The parents return home with an agreement that their children are never to know where they went. Clearly, this approach shouldn't be used if it leaves younger children at the mercy of a potentially violent adolescent. However, it's been known to help shift the balance of power and to restore power to parents. Some parents of aggressive young people care too much about their children's feelings and would never do anything their children might find painful, like the Palazzoli technique; they usually react with feelings of guilt. If parents can be influenced to go away, as prescribed in the Palazzoli technique, their children may be so shocked that they will rethink their entire attitude of frightening their parents into submission. If parents can differentiate themselves from their children enough to take a step as powerful as Palazzoli's, there's no telling what else they might get together and do.

Another adult who is there to help provide physical control of an adolescent and protection for other family members may need to be moved into the house. As in the case of an adolescent with Level 4 aggression, it's preferable if parents don't use the authorities. However, a visit by the police, a petition in juvenile court, or a night spent at the juvenile detention facility or in jail may be a real eye-opener for an adolescent and may force him or her to reconsider embarking on a life of crime. A short time spent with those who truly qualify as criminals may help teenagers recognize that they aren't as tough as they thought.

STOPPING SERIOUS DANGER AND HARM: INTERVENTION AT LEVEL 6

How to intervene in a case of serious physical violence must be carefully considered. An everyday experience provided me with some sage advice that metaphorically applies to the dilemma of intervening in violence: On his 7th birthday our eldest son, Joshua, was given the gift of a hamster he could pick out at the store. When Joshua was presented with a large cage full of hamsters to choose from, we asked the store owner how he could choose a good hamster. He suggested that I reach in and grab one; if it bit me, we shouldn't buy that one. I wasn't thrilled with this rather risky recommendation. After Josh had decided on a hamster he liked, I again asked the store owner's advice. This time I asked him how to get the chosen hamster out of its cage. I'd hoped that he would offer to transfer the animal to our cage for us, but I was disappointed. However, the advice he gave me was worth the risk of hamster bite: "Reach in fast, grab it firmly, and get it out quick. If you hesitate or pull your hand back, he'll bite you."

The advice I offer parents of adolescents at Level 6 aggression is similar: One can't afford to act hesitantly with someone who might become violent. It's better that parents not intervene at all unless they're prepared to act with confidence. Approaches at Level 6 include techniques that involve people outside the family. Moving outsiders into the home, even when violence has already reached Level 6, may succeed in disrupting the violence. The Palazzoli prescription continues to be powerful at this stage. Because it removes the intended victims (in that the parents are asked to leave), this prescription may be wiser than strategies that encourage parents to go head-to-head with a violent teenager or young adult.

Techniques designed to benevolently disrupt violent behavior have to be used with caution. Parents could do something kind that's intended to calm things down and, instead, end up antagonizing their teenager into an outburst that could get someone killed. The therapist must explore all past patterns of interaction that have led to violent outbursts before prescribing a course of action. Parents commonly give oversimplified answers when the therapist requests information about the circumstances surrounding incidents of violence. They'll say, "He just explodes, and there's nothing we can do," or "I just look at him the wrong way, and he starts swearing at me." The therapist must clearly understand the atmosphere of the household at the time of a violent incident, the preceding actions of the adolescent, the types of parental responses that have brought about dangerous explosions, and parental approaches that are just plain antagonistic. Interactional patterns always exist that, if understood, can give the therapist ideas about approaches that aren't dangerous and haven't been tried. Parents who live in a fearful fog that leads them to generalize about their child must be led through a step-by-step interactional assessment of what happens at home. Parents who are constantly angry tend to generalize, as do those who have become sullenly immune to abuse by their children.

Explorations into the family system to access more information will test how workable the situation is. Strategies by the therapist should be basically benevolent ones that remove the victims from potential violence. If improvement doesn't happen through benevolent acts, then the powerful, carefully planned decisive steps previously discussed are the next directions to pursue. Tough love approaches that are designed to expel the young person from the home presuppose that the parents have the wherewithal to enforce such a decision. In cases of violence, expelling a child from the home may lead to someone getting hurt unless plans are made to ensure everyone's protection and all contingencies are anticipated and responses to them are prepared thoroughly. In addition, the adolescent may not have the slightest ability to live on his or her own and could meet with a horrible fate.

As with Level 5, Level 6 may signal the time to accept that force (in the form of restraint) or the authorities must be used. Again, such decisive action can't be done hesitantly. An adolescent confronted at home by police is likely to become even more dangerous to the family after the police leave unless the police involvement is a powerful and frightening experience. If police are called, parents have to be prepared to have their son or daughter arrested and to press charges. Empty threats by parents are experienced by teenagers with Level 6 aggression as laughable, and hesitant attempts to intervene physically are like pulling your hand back when reaching into a cage of hamsters. Pulling back will result in getting bitten. Whatever the action, parents should be helped to develop contingency plans to provide protection for themselves in case of retaliation.

As you can see, assessing aggressive and violent adolescents accurately is a complicated process. The actions therapists must take, once the case is properly assessed, are direct and often frightening. Despite the dangerous waters therapists are wading through in such cases, they must be flexible enough to look at the unique features of each situation, determine what must be done, and influence those involved to act decisively.

Perhaps the greatest challenge to therapists is to make the transition from identifying what the problem is to deciding on a strategy or approach that makes sense in light of the assessment. Such a bridge between assessment and intervention is explored in the next chapter by looking at the ancient Chinese philosophy of Taoism and how the *Tao Te Ching* can direct therapists to simple yet powerful ways of thinking and acting.

SEVEN

The Tao of Family Therapy

A Strategy for Treating Adolescents with Psychiatric Symptoms

The more laws and restrictions there are,
The poorer people become.
The sharper men's weapons,
The more trouble in the land.
The more ingenious and clever men are,
The more strange things happen.

      —LAO TSU (*Tao Te Ching*,
      Chap. 57)

The speed with which master therapists move from limited information to strategies for change is always startling. Whether they know it or not, these masters have an understanding of people that directs them toward an economical way of organizing what they see in a first session. This chapter offers therapists a method for orienting themselves to see the central interaction that's paralyzing a family struggling with an abusive adolescent and for then nudging that interaction in such a way that new options, behaviors, and relationships emerge.

A view of human relations exists that can transform what has become known as resistance into flexibility and a greater ability to change. This philosophy encapsulates human nature and directs the natural impulses and drives of humans in such a way that many of the pitfalls in human problem solving can be avoided. Any theory that presents an approach for dealing with psychiatric symptoms in abusive young people must be specific to the individual's unique situation, yet this same theory should stimulate therapists to develop ideas about how the approach can be applied to a range of mental health problems. Many writers have made attempts to capture the essence of movement in therapy in a manner that makes creating change at once spontaneous and reproducible.

Salvador Minuchin and Charles Fishman (1981) addressed the question of therapeutic spontaneity by likening the position of the therapist to that of a Japanese samurai who becomes one with his opponent in order to overcome him. These therapists advise their readers to read their book and then give it away and forget having read it. Donald Saposnek (1980) explores strategic therapy from the perspective of its likeness to aikido. A practitioner of the martial art of aikido approaches a challenge by joining with the position of an opponent. Rather than attack a problem the way karate or confrontational therapies do, aikido uses the momentum created by the opponent to transform his aggression into cooperation. As it is with the abstract principle of therapeutic spontaneity, the ability to productively use resistance in treatment is a hard skill to teach.

Philosophies that use Oriental wisdom to guide therapy can be most easily understood by returning to an early source from which Oriental teachings arose. One has only to begin exploring aikido to notice that the philosophy underlying this martial art must have arisen from the teachings of the *Tao Te Ching*.

Approximately 2,500 years ago a great Chinese sage named Lao Tsu wrote one of the most widely translated texts in history. The Tao is best translated as "The Way." According to an Oriental tale reported by Jacob Needleman (cited in Lao Tsu, 1989):

> Confucius once journeyed to see Lao Tsu and came away amazed and in awe of the man. According to the tale, Confucius described his meeting with Lao Tsu in the following way. "I know a bird can fly, a fish can swim, an animal can run. For that which runs a net can be made; for that which swims a line can be made; for that which flies a corded arrow can be made. But the dragon's ascent into heaven on the wind and the clouds is something which is beyond my knowledge. Today I have seen Lao Tsu who is perhaps like a dragon." (p. vii)

What is there about the teachings of Lao Tsu that made even Confucius stand in awe? The *Tao Te Ching* is made up of brief, somewhat abstract statements that are meant to elicit responses on a deep level. Any attempt to offer a circumscribed meaning to the Tao ultimately ends fruitlessly. Many find meanings for themselves but consensus can never be reached. The writings of the Tao appear to be intended as triggers that lead the student spontaneously to a higher state of consciousness and life. By definition, if readers believe they have completely grasped the Tao, full understanding has eluded them. The very act of thinking one knows everything makes it impossible for one to understand.

This paradox about knowing the Tao resembles techniques used in strategic therapy. Strategies are intended to spontaneously unleash the potential in families to change and heal their hurts. If those who are receiving therapy become preoccupied with insight and obsessed with understanding, their ability to live life in a new and more evolved way may elude them. Change occurs when the actions of a therapist can lead clients to simply do what's needed. Therapy often succeeds to whatever extent clients take action while being mindless of the underlying intent. In Chapter 22 of the *Tao Te Ching*, Lao Tsu states:

> Yield and overcome;
> Bend and be straight;
> Empty and be full;
> Wear out and be new;
> Have little and gain;
> Have much and be confused.

The more numerous the complex theories, understandings, diagnostics, and definitions therapists are encumbered with, the more helpless they become to bring about change. Therapists can be blinded by manufactured concepts. People are no longer seen as people, no longer understood as unique beings existing in a unique context. The content blinds the therapist to the process. In Chapter 5 of the *Tao Te Ching*, Lao Tsu states:

> Heaven and earth are impartial;
> They see the ten thousand things as straw dogs;
> The wise are impartial;
> They see the people as straw dogs;
>
> The space between heaven and earth is like a bellows;
> The shape changes but not the form;
> The more it moves, the more it yields;
> More words count less;
> Hold fast to the center.

Lao Tsu is advising the reader to seek balance. Reality is elusive when viewed through the lens of any given moment, so one must step back and get a larger sense of the context of a problem. People must not be deceived by words when their experience and inner guidance disagree with those words. The challenge is to understand how to hold on to that center.

When experienced therapists or supervisors are asked why they chose to move in a certain clinical direction at a certain time, they typically reflect for a long time before answering. After reflection those masters will often simply say that it seemed like the right thing to do at the time. Great therapists spend many years seeing families and studying the lore and craft of therapy until they can trust their unconscious minds to give them answers without having to seek them. How does a therapist grasp what those right things are without spending 10 or 15 years treating families? How do they learn to stop being misled by feelings and opinions? One way to speed up the process of being able to trust one's unconscious is found in the Tao.

The emotional abuse dished out by aggressive adolescents with psychiatric symptoms is different enough from other emotionally abusive behaviors to warrant separate handling. It is the one form of abuse parents are sympathetic to because they don't identify it as abuse. When an emotionally distressed teenager enters the psychiatric system, that system then cooperates in the abuse of the parents by diagnosing the young person as mentally ill and, often, by blaming the parents. The label of mental illness takes an adolescent's symptoms out of the realm of problems parents feel qualified to deal with. Parents are often left helplessly at the sidelines as they watch their child deteriorate through repeated hospitalizations and different medications. The removal of the parents' authority and expertise is the largest single factor that puts abusive power into a child's hands.

WHO IS IN CONTROL?

Cloé Madanes (1981) discussed "power balancing in couples" as a process by which the least powerful person in a relationship becomes symptomatic. As the "healthy" and more powerful spouse tries to help the mate resolve these symptoms, the latter sees to it that all attempts to help fail. This refusal to be helped successfully removes power from the hands of the stronger spouse and puts so much power back in the hands of the weaker one that the power is equalized between them. The only problem with this solution is that the troubled spouse must remain forever troubled to maintain this balance. A perfect example is that of an affair. Who's the stronger party in a marriage where one spouse is unfaithful? It would seem that the one having the affair is in charge since he or she has made a choice and is acting on it. Yet why would a powerful person need to sneak around as if fearful of incurring the wrath of others when found out? The choice of an affair is an act that gains needed power for the unfaithful spouse. A person who's weak enough to begin an affair may feel more powerful in relationship to the spouse once the affair is under way. He or she feels more loved and appreciated by the lover, which improves self-esteem.

Such a power imbalance exists when young people use psychiatric symptoms to abuse their parents (Madanes, 1981). Ideally, both partners in a marriage are equal but a natural hierarchy exists between parents and children. However, troubled teenagers tend to see themselves as equals to their parents, even though society restricts the rights, and therefore the power of minors. Knowing that their power is unequal to their parents' many troubled adolescents attempt to enhance their power by becoming symptomatic. Any therapist who has worked with a family in which a child has been diagnosed with a serious mental disease and medicated has experienced the helplessness and loss of control that parents feel. Parents describe feeling as if they've lost their son or daughter, as if they no longer know who their child is. It would be difficult to find a more effective method for bringing parents down several notches on the power continuum than to diagnose their child as mentally ill. The adults involved then move into predictable patterns of behavior that the child can manipulate by demonstrating specific symptoms at specific times. Because the child appears to be a helpless victim of an overwhelming disease and because the parents fear that they would feel even guiltier than they already do if they try to put pressure on a helpless victim of a disease, the parents' attempts to take charge are usually ineffectual and short-lived.

Evan was a 15-year-old boy who'd been diagnosed as manic–depressive. He had unpredictable outbursts of temper and would attack other children. Knowing he had a disease frightened school personnel; therefore, they hesitated to suspend Evan or use punishments they freely used with other students who acted the same way. When Evan told a teacher to "fuck off" and walked out of class, he was "punished" by having to talk to the school counselor. He was further "punished" by being given a pass he could use to leave class and go to the counselor's office whenever he found it difficult to "deal with the stress." Evan gained incredible power over his teachers and school administrators by acts of aggression and bizarre behavior. For example, whenever he began to gesture or talk in disconnected ways, his teachers would become terrified of the threat of a full-blown manic episode in their classes and would then reduce their demands on Evan because the psychiatrist had said that he couldn't handle too much pressure. Furthermore, after the doctor told Evan's parents that manic–depressive illness was genetic, the parents engaged in convoluted discussions about whether or not Evan was responsible for his actions. The doctor's diagnosis also made them wonder which of them had passed this plague on to their son, so they felt guilty and confused when trying to decide what action to take. When deciding on consequences, Evan's parents would argue endlessly over the pros and cons of harshness versus permissiveness.

The pattern of abuse by psychiatric symptoms is seen in adolescents who feel powerless to change family problems they find painful to be around. For example, parents may be harsh, rigid, and ineffectual in their child-rearing efforts, or other children in the house may be mishandled. These disturbed adolescents have found that direct methods of confronting problems in the family are rapidly blocked. In order to make their parents take notice of their transgressions (whether real or not), children become troubled and, by doing so, force their parents to become active in resolving the concerns. Some parents are then able to focus on their children in new ways and take charge of solving the problems; in such cases the adolescent's symptoms resolve themselves. However, this success can occur only if the parents confront the situation effectively before serious psychiatric intervention takes the handling of the problem out of their hands.

More serious problems happen when parents refuse to make the connection between their children's symptoms and other family problems. What began as an attempted solution then takes on the function of punishing parents for their transgressions and for their refusal to see that they've mishandled things. Adolescents keep the power they've gained by being disturbed and, as time passes, experience extensive secondary gain. For example, they're excused from fulfilling age-appropriate responsibilities and receive help and solicitous gestures from parents and other adults; they may even experience affection from their parents, which had stopped before their symptoms emerged.

Having serious psychiatric symptoms becomes a successful way of organizing daily existence. These troubled adolescents have created a new way of living that never has to change, even as they continue to punish their parents most cruelly for their transgressions and mishandling of the family. As the adolescent's troubled behavior continues, the parents feel more disheartened and guilty about the plight of their children, especially if the child was close to one or both of them before the problems began. Typically, adolescents won't relinquish the power they've gained, because the new balance that has been reached has stopped what they saw as their parents' misuse of power. These children find that they now have as much power as their parents do—and in some cases even more. A troubled adolescent punishes parents by making them watch his or her suffering and deterioration, an exercise that keeps a power balance the adolescent is in control of. He or she can escalate symptoms any time the parents are suspected of gaining or misusing their power.

ADOLESCENTS IN THE FAMILY CONTEXT

Abusive adolescents with psychiatric symptoms offer us a proving ground for working with the approach that has grown out of Taoist philosophy. We will develop a model for looking at family dilemmas and at young people who present chronic psychiatric symptoms, rather than get buried in what the problems seem to be. Families already know what their problems seem to be but can't find solutions. With this new clinical perspective, the therapist identifies simply understood struggles in the client family and begins from that point rather than become embroiled in the same convoluted drama the family is already caught in (Price, 1988). The therapist must be as much like *P'u*, which translates as "the uncarved block," as possible (Hoff, 1982). This Chinese word, which can be thought of as synonymous with words like *natural, simple, plain,* or *honest,* suggests movement back toward the most simple, original, and uncompromised form a human being can take in approaching a situation.

For several years I've been showing a videotape of a segment from the classic Disney movie of A. A. Milne's "Winnie the Pooh and Tigger Too" to illustrate how to think simply and straightforwardly about a problem. I learned later that Benjamin Hoff, the author of *The Tao of Pooh* (1982), uses the same segment from Milne's book to illustrate the concept of *P'u*. A. A. Milne created a namesake for an ancient Chinese philosophical concept, along with other characters that dramatize the essence of Taoism. Following the example of Winnie the Pooh, "a bear of very little brain," the therapist must be like *P'u*, the uncarved block. How does a therapist simplify and understand the problem a child or adolescent is experiencing? *P'u* directs the therapist back to the point in time when the child's problems began, back to the moment in the young person's development that his or her behavior is directing everyone to look at.

Such a simplistic way of viewing problems can best be described as *seeing things for what they are* rather than defining them in more and more complicated ways. Experience suggests that once a situation has been described in terms derived from how people are actually interacting, ideas naturally generate themselves to guide the therapist toward the proper steps for changing the rigidly embedded problematic situation. When working with abusive teenagers who have psychiatric symptoms, how can the therapist think like Pooh (or is it *P'u*?)? The answers to the following questions can guide the therapist toward accomplishing this difficult task:

1. What stage of the family's life cycle or the child's development do family members believe they are in? (This is the apparent age in relationship.)

    Example: Parents act as if their 20-year-old son is a capable adult who should be treated as such. By waiting for spontaneous action and not intervening directly, they continue, fruitlessly, to attempt to get him to decide to take responsibility for himself. They often say "We can't make him do what he should" or "He has to do it for himself."

2. What level of the family's development is the symptomatic person operating at? (This is the actual age in relationship.)

    Example: The aforementioned 20-year-old expects to stay home indefinitely at no charge, be given money, not have to work, and not be inconvenienced by his parents. At what age does a young person live such a life?

3. Now attach an age to each level: (a) What age are the parents acting as if the child is? and (b) What age does the child behave as if he or she is?

    For example:

    Apparent age in relationship (often the same as biological age): 20 years old

    Actual age in relationship (when looked at based on behavior): 13 years old

4. If the young adult were actually the age his or her behavior suggests, how would the parents be advised to act in relationship to their child?

5. How could the situation be arranged so that it mimics the actual age in the relationship?

    Example: The parents in our example could be advised by the therapist to negotiate an arrangement in which their son, in order to continue to receive room, board, and money, must agree to allow them to take charge of his search for a job. Such an agreement could require the parents to schedule their son's time, take him to fill out employment applications, instruct him on how to dress, and show him how to manage money responsibly, much as they would handle a 13-year-old. Many people believe that a power struggle between parents and a young adult, like this 20-year-old, is the result of attempts on the parents' part to treat the young adult like a much younger child, which in turn encourages the young person to act like one. Such parents actually treat their child like a 13-year-old emotionally but still expect him or her to take on a 20-year-old's responsibilities. For instance, they'll read the young adult's mail and then scold him or her for not paying a bill. A Tao-based treatment process would arrange for the young person's emotional and behavioral functioning to be congruent. Therefore, if parents read their child's mail, they'd also be responsible for helping pay the child's bills or for educating him or her about how to do so. By the same token, if parents think their son or daughter should be totally responsible for bill paying, they would respect the young adult's privacy and leave his or her mail unopened.

6. As the behavior of the young person begins to more closely resemble that of a responsible person of the same age, how can the interaction between parents and young adult be modified to more closely resemble the young person's biological age?

In the following example the clarification of incongruent responses by family members was crucial in solving the problem of an adolescent with serious psychosomatic symptoms.

CLINICAL VIGNETTE: THE HELPFUL BROTHER

Thirteen-year-old Ken, who lived in rural northern Michigan, was brought for private therapy by his parents, who were both professionals. He was slightly overweight and had a sallow complexion, and his dark hair looked as if it hadn't been washed for a week. Ken had been suffering from chronic stomachaches, headaches, and weakness, a condition for which doctors hadn't been able to find a medical cause. By the pained expressions on his parents' faces and the matter-of-fact look on Ken's, I had an immediate impression that for some reason Ken was tormenting his parents by making them watch him slowly destroy his life.

Ken hadn't been in school for over a year, rarely left the house, never saw his old friends, and isolated himself in his bedroom to watch television. During the interview I didn't learn anything that explained why Ken might be having these problems. His mother's response to him vacillated between compassionate support and a rage that erupted whenever she admitted to herself that her maternal efforts failed to comfort her son and ease his pain. His father swung back and forth between anger at his wife for not standing up to Ken and withdrawal when he saw her raging at Ken. Despite their troubled interaction around Ken's symptoms, his parents appeared to be independent people who loved each other and weren't demonstrating symptoms that could explain why their son would be worried enough to give up his adolescence and stay home to watch over things. That is, Ken's parents appeared to have a loving relationship that didn't require a third party to stabilize it.

Ken had been a good student and had had many friends at school before becoming homebound. There didn't seem to be any reason for him to avoid school because of problems at home. It was reasonable to assume, though, that he would have some difficulty stepping back into a normal school routine after being away for so many months and falling, academically and emotionally, behind his classmates.

Despite the temptation to focus on Ken's emotional conflicts, I decided that it was better to begin by working directly on what could be done to get him back to a normal routine. Ken's parents had already done many appropriate things to help him, but each time he began to make progress, his symptoms would become more extreme. When he tried to go out, Ken had more pain and fears than when he sat safely in his room. His parents would then be faced with a power struggle they could only win by resorting to a high level of force and actions that seemed cruel to them. Powerful action, such as physically removing Ken from his room and taking him to school, was difficult for these parents who loved their suffering son dearly.

I began the interview by asking Ken's parents to describe behavior they considered to be typical of a healthy 13-year-old boy. They made a list of behaviors that included the following:

- Attends school regularly.
- Does things outside the house with friends.
- Helps around the house with chores.
- Makes some independent decisions wisely.
- Keeps his own room reasonably neat.
- Spends time when at home both alone in his room and with the family.
- Participates in most family activities.
- Dresses himself and picks his own clothes.
- Puts dirty clothes in the hamper to be washed.
- Gets to sleep at a reasonable hour.

We then discussed behavioral details that focused on level of responsibility, independent action, and self-regulation. Once this list was completed, we discussed Ken's current behaviors in these areas and the age level indicated by those behaviors. They made the following list:

- Ken wasn't in school, so his academic age couldn't be set at an age older than 5.

◆ Ken hadn't left the house alone in many months, a behavior typical of a preschool-age child.

◆ Ken's way of complaining and whining about his symptoms resembled the behavior of children 5 to 7 years old.

◆ Ken didn't go out with friends and none came over to his house, the typical situation for a 2- or 3-year-old.

◆ Ken often didn't get dressed at all during the day but remained in his pajamas, like an infant.

◆ Ken complained about going to bed at night and kept coming out of his room, like children 4 to 8 years old.

◆ Ken wanted to be seen in treatment without his family. This was typical behavior for a 13-year-old; adolescents usually complain about the presence of their parents in the therapy room and want the therapist for a confidant.

◆ Ken rarely spoke back to his parents. Although they preferred this aspect of his current condition, they were willing to agree that few children over the age of 5 or 6 are this agreeable.

Because Ken's parents and I agreed that his behaviors pointed to an actual age in relationship of 5, I described his problem as an unexplained developmental lag. I then asked the parents how they would behave toward a 5-year-old son and how this behavior would be different from the actions of a 13-year-old's parents. Ken willingly participated in this discussion. The following is a list of many of the points that were agreed on:

◆ Parents of a 5-year-old would expect very little independent behavior in the child and wouldn't respond angrily when such behavior wasn't forthcoming.

◆ The parents of a 5-year-old boy would be very protective; that is, they would monitor his food intake and nutrition closely, hold his hand as they crossed the street, cut meat for him, and so forth.

◆ A 5-year-old would have television content monitored closely because young children are very impressionable.

◆ Parents would make sure that a 5-year-old gets a lot of hugs and reassurance.

◆ Parents would establish a bedtime appropriate for a 5-year-old, would make sure their child was tucked in properly at night, and would read him a bedtime story.

◆ Parents would decide whether or not their 5-year-old would get dressed, when he would dress, and what he would wear.

Before coming to therapy Ken's parents were treating him like a 5-year-old while acting as if they expected him to behave like a 13-year-old. They would then become angry when he continued to act like a 5-year-old. This incongruity between how family members act and how they conceptualize themselves acting is frequently evident when adolescents have psychiatric symptoms. The simultaneous existence of two incompatible frames of reference characterizes the emotional paralysis that stymies change. Change becomes possible only when the family is helped into a single frame of reference.

Many therapists prefer an approach that isolates one frame of reference by utilizing a "tough love" philosophy to force children to "grow up" and act their age. This approach is anything but loving and ignores the important fact that there's a reason for the young person's immature behavior. The tough love approach doesn't create an opportunity for less severely disturbed young people to work out important issues within themselves or with their families. Asking the family to act in ways consistent with the child's actual age in relationship enables parents and teenagers to look closely at how they wish to live and permits them to move forward one step at a time toward a relationship that's consistent with the child's biological age.

Surprisingly, Ken seemed eager for the activity of the upcoming week. His interest suggested that a higher level of expressed love and devotion from his parents was what he was trying to achieve by creating his symptoms. Ken would have resisted the approach I was suggesting had he truly wanted his parents to be less intrusive. He just wanted them to be less angry.

The next week was spent implementing the agreed-upon plan to establish a lifestyle based on the agreements reached that were consistent with Ken's actual age in relationship. At the second session I moved the discussion immediately to how that plan was implemented and how his parents would now assess the age level he was operating at. His parents felt that Ken had progressed to 6 or 7 years old because he was going outside the house alone. As his parents continued to both pamper and restrict him, based on the new age of 7, Ken began to leave his room and stopped complaining about his stomach, head, and lethargy. When he seemed more normal, his parents began to feel comfortable putting pressure on him to attend school. Within a month of the implementation of our strategy, Ken was back in school. I spent a lot of time collaborating with school personnel to help ease Ken back into a normal academic routine.

Readers may find themselves thinking, "That seems too easy. What's the catch?" In fact, there was a catch. Once Ken was back in school and had "grown" from a 5-year-old to a 13-year-old, he began to act like a teenager in other ways. He became more verbally aggressive and opposed his parents in ways that mortified them. The more rigid they became in response to his behavior, the more oppositional he became. Ken's new behavior upset them so much that they threatened to expel him from the house and the family. The parents' difficulty in dealing with Ken's adolescence began to make explicit what it was about their handling of the family that he was punishing them for. It turned out that shortly before Ken began to have problems, his 19-year-old sister, who they had never mentioned, and with whom he was very close, had moved out of the house to get married. Ken's mother didn't approve of her choice and had screamed and fought with her terribly. When screaming and arguing didn't work, Ken's mother ostracized her daughter from the family. She had barely spoken to her since. Ken's parents were so sweet and loving that they had no tolerance for the push and pull that's normal with adolescents. Ken knew his parents could more easily handle his apparent medical symptoms than his attempts to grow up and resist their control. After all, they'd already handled his sister's rebelliousness poorly.

There was still therapy to be done in teaching Ken and his parents how to negotiate and in showing his parents how to move into a new stage of life with both children. Through the use of a Taoist philosophy I was able to move this case, in which a young adolescent had at first used psychiatric symptoms to abuse his parents, into a range of disturbance any competent therapist would know what to do with.

Although this approach can be used when a child's psychiatric symptoms have little to do with difficulty in a family relationship, a Taoist approach can also be used when an individual adult's psychiatric symptoms develop for other reasons. People with fears may develop symptoms designed to avoid a feared situation. Again, an incongruity may be shown to exist between how people view themselves and how they're actually living their lives as the result of a symptom. People may avoid their worst fears and simultaneously live as if the feared situation has already occurred. Using a Taoist philosophy, the therapist—as the uncarved block—recognizes the way clients have come to live their lives instead of being fooled by his or her own cleverness in interpreting individual symptoms.

CLINICAL VIGNETTE: USING A TAO-BASED APPROACH WITH A YOUNG ADULT

Although not an adolescent case, the following example demonstrates the treatment incongruity, which, though no longer directed at parents, began there. If her condition were to deteriorate this client could well find herself back at home being taken care of by her parents. Many late adolescents seek therapy with similar symptoms.

Jeanine was a 24-year-old woman with a beautiful head of flaming red hair. She had recently finished college, had moved into her own apartment, and had begun teaching first grade. However, she was having terrible fears that she was losing her hair. She constantly worried about the prospect of having to wear a wig and losing her womanhood. Each day Jeanine would wake up and count the hairs on her pillow and chart the pattern of hair loss. As she became consumed by her fear that her hair loss already showed, Jeanine limited her activities outside her home to the point where she only left her apartment to go to work.

Jeanine had seen a number of doctors and psychiatrists, who had given her various medications and had run numerous tests. Although she was losing a bit more hair than normal, Jeanine looked perfectly fine. None of the doctors could find anything wrong with her; they considered the marginal hair loss to be due to stress and depression. To any uninformed observer Jeanine appeared to have a lovely head of hair (and certainly enough hair to make a bald writer of therapy articles incredibly envious). Yet she was living as if she'd already lost her hair. If Jeanine had truly lost her hair, her anxiety and isolation would have been exactly the same as she was imposing on herself now and she would have had no social life or dates (as was the case at the time of the interview). Jeanine was isolating herself as thoroughly as if she had lost her hair and were hiding herself out of embarrassment over having to wear a wig.

The therapist's job in this case, as it was with Ken, was to do away with the incongruity that was keeping the client emotionally paralyzed. To make the problem more congruent, the therapist prescribed the completion of the reality that Jeanine had created for herself. She was directed to begin shopping for a wig. The condition that she had created for herself implicitly was made explicit, as it was with Ken; this was so that Jeanine could make a real choice between being devastated by her fear of hair loss or approaching her situation more reasonably.

The Tao-based approach confronts people with the reality they've created for themselves; the world is then allowed to respond to them as if their internally produced reality had become external reality. In the case of Jeanine's self-abuse, it was never known who or what she was responding to, but her situation had the characteristics of a case where psychiatric symptoms were being used to abuse someone. Once Jeanine was offered the chance to pursue her fears, she began seeing her hair loss in a balanced way and gradually returned to normal activities. Her fear became a conscious choice rather than an involuntary reaction.

CONCLUSION

The dilemma of incongruity between the relationships people would be having based on their biological age and those they are having based on their actual age in relationship is seen in a large percentage of therapy cases. Therapists tend toward handling the situation through one or the other frame of reference. They tend to either emphasize the need to resolve the past or concentrate primarily on what needs to be changed in the present. Understanding the incongruity involved and treating the situation with both frames of reference in mind enlarges the therapist's view of the situation so that he or she can address the confusion that typifies the emotional world of both client and family. Such an approach reduces fear and emotional paralysis in clients as they try to understand these symptoms that make them feel as if they're lost.

Jay Haley (1980) identified the stage of leaving home as a common time at which symptoms such as psychosis and major depression emerge. Many states of internal confusion can be explained by the fact that the person is facing the dilemma of choosing in which world to live. Both identified client and family move freely back and forth between a relationship based on the identified client's biological age and actual age in relationship with no set pattern emerging for the therapist to grasp hold of and treat.

The discrepancy caused by movement between incongruent states of mind and interaction also plague adult survivors of childhood incest; they can't decide if they're childhood victim or family stabilizer (Deighton & McPeek, 1985). Are they victimized children responding to powerful parents, or are they adults dealing with memories of past indiscretions by aging or now dead parents? Rampant incongruity brings about memory loss or pseudopsychotic symptoms to resolve that incongruity. Therapy reorganizes the situation hierarchically, so the set of incongruous relationships once again align and make sense (Madanes, 1990). Once proper restitution and healthy relationships are restored, there's no one left to be victimized.

The *Tao Te Ching* provides a simple and practical set of guidelines for bringing about realignment of incongruent relationship patterns. Both worlds—what people are doing and what they're acting as if they're doing—are real, and both must be addressed. The aggressor who wishes to attack must be brought into alignment with the Tao-based defender, who wishes to resolve the dilemma without violence or assault. Therapists can understand and join with the reality of the families they're working with. By accepting a family's view of the world, the therapist becomes a trusted guide and is able to bring the family's incongruous realities back into line with reality while exposing other issues in need of treatment and doing away with the need for further symptoms.

A new problem emerges, though, when adolescents are acting dangerously and threatening violence. The art of directive therapy requires that therapists have an extensive repertoire of methods for helping people change their lives and for alleviating their symptoms. When the symptom is overt aggression rather than anxiety or depression, therapists must help families take immediate powerful measures to block the possibility of violence. In the next chapter therapists are guided through a variety of steps they can help parents take to fight fire with fire by using the power of conspiracy and collusion as a secret weapon.

EIGHT

The Secret
Weapon Strategy
Conspiracy and
Collusion in Therapy

The problem of potentially violent adolescents has plagued therapists for as long as there has been treatment for teenagers. Traditional approaches often employ psychodynamic individual therapies or utilize agents of social control, such as juvenile court and police, in place of a more active and directive counseling. Nondirective psychodynamic approaches that focus on feelings break down when adolescents threaten violence. Adolescents have the power to stop therapy in its tracks by being openly aggressive or threatening to harm someone. Although some of these teenagers have proven themselves to be dangerous, the majority are dramatic actors whose menacing role of villainy parents and professionals alike find highly threatening. With the smallest of acts these angry, threatening adolescents create a sinister cloud that follows them everywhere.

The power adolescents use may be blatant and openly abusive. Their assaults may be disguised as convincing discourse that pokes holes through parents' self-confidence until they can no longer hold ground and act with decision. Robert Boswell, in his novel *Mystery Ride* (1992), offers a fictional account of the subtle use of power by a teenager. Dulcie, a 15-year-old, and her mother, Angela, are in the car. Angela is taking Dulcie to the country to stay with her father in hopes that rural life will help her get her behavior back in line. Angela is trying to connect with her daughter in a conversational way (pp. 65–66).

Dulcie returned with a six-pack of Diet Pepsi. "Isn't it kind of early for that?" Angela asked.

"It's too early for anything, we're here, aren't we?" Dulcie popped open a can. Angela steered them back onto the freeway.

"The artificial sweetener in that—" Angela indicated the Pepsi "—may not be entirely safe. Some doctors don't recommend it for children under fourteen or pregnant women."

"If this is your clever way of asking me if I'm pregnant, I'm not."

"I was doing no such thing," Angela said, although she felt a small wave of relief. "I just thought we could talk about something. I happen to know that sweetener has an odd history in getting its approval from the FDA."

"This is supposed to interest me?"

"You pick a subject."

"How about the way you're running my life by making me spend the whole summer in Cowtown, Iowa?"

"You're spending the summer with your father. You've always liked going to the farm."

"Not for the whole summer."

"Well, you'll have to make the best of it. Your father loves you and he doesn't get to see that much of you."

"You're sending me there to punish me, and you know it."

"I'm taking you to the place you were born to spend the summer with your father." Angela said this angrily, then forced herself to continue in order to admit the whole truth. "And, yes, I think it would be good for you to get away from those so-called friends of yours."

"So I've heard about a thousand times now." With a long gulp, she finished her first Diet Pepsi and popped open a second. "You think your friends are so great? You think anybody would ever want to wind up like one of you? If you're willing to talk, talk, talk about politics, that's all you have to do to be one of your friends."

"A lot of people I loathe talk about politics all the time," Angela said, aware that she wasn't really defending herself or her friends very well.

"So? They're just on the wrong side. If they would jump over to your side, they'd become your friends. Even if they were push-button freaks."

This conversation has a quality that's prevalent in discussions with aggressive teenagers. Despite Angela's numerous attempts to take charge of the situation and generate a discussion that would be pleasant and companionable, Dulcie winds up in charge. Without realizing how, Angela finds herself reacting to Dulcie rather than the other way around. Angela is the parent, yet she's defending herself without knowing how she got into a struggle. Dulcie calls the shots.

Teenagers and young adults who wield power challenge us to understand the nature of power in relationships. When that power becomes destructive, we're further challenged to expand our understanding of the reasons for young people's aggressive behavior and of the techniques therapists can use to help them improve. Where does adolescent power come from? What's happening when parents and professionals fail to keep explosive teens under control?

In our world it's clear that information is power. Education, libraries, computers, and other sources of information hold the keys to understanding and controlling our world. Knowledge passed from person to person has always held the key to conquering and taming our environment. How do aggressive adolescents harness the power of information in such a way that they keep their parents in thrall and make them feel incapable of regaining control?

If information is power, it stands to reason that whoever's in control of the flow of information will prevail. In war, the country with the best intelligence system is likely to win regardless of firepower. In the Vietnam War the North Vietnamese prevailed over American troops because they knew where the Americans were at any given time and because their style of guerrilla warfare kept American troops wondering where they were going to be assaulted from next. In addition, the North Vietnamese used booby traps as a way of whittling away at the enemy; booby traps are effective weapons because only those who set them have the information necessary to avoid them. Thus, despite significantly fewer soldiers and much less firepower, the North Vietnamese ultimately drove the American troops out of Vietnam.

Guerrilla warfare is in many ways akin to the tactics used by abusive young people. Adolescents use a variety of techniques that help ensure their access to information about the lives of adults, but they're guarded when disclosing information about themselves and their comings and goings. Teenagers often conspire with others to limit their parents' access to information about their activities. Adolescents seek out counselors and other sympathetic adults who'll collude with them against their parents by refusing to share with the parents information about their activities and concerns. Aggressive teenagers choose friends whose parents are somewhat adolescent themselves. Emotionally adolescent adults are more likely to keep the confidences of a teenager regardless of the seriousness of the young person's behavior.

Therapists as a group are a fairly moralistic bunch who consider themselves above using the time-honored methods employed by their teenage clients for bringing about change. Many new therapists touting the language of solution-focused therapy (O'Hanlon & Weiner-Davis, 1989; de Shazer, 1985), reflecting teams (Andersen, 1991), or conversational approaches proclaim the need for a "collaborative" approach to therapy. They talk about the need to learn what works to bring about change from our clients. The primary difference between solution-focused approaches and the strategic approach put forth in this book has to do with hierarchy.

In his earliest book Haley (1964) made the following point, which came out of his focus on communication: All interaction between humans can be understood as a series of maneuvers; that is, whether consciously or unconsciously, people are always trying to influence each other. Therefore, therapy should be the conscious use of the therapist's skills to influence clients toward change. This view, common among strategists, necessarily involves defining a role in which therapists are hierarchically above clients. That is to say, therapists are in charge and have the responsibility for identifying the nature of a troubled interaction and for devising a solution.

The up-and-coming approaches are more accurately described as collaborative, nonauthoritarian models of family therapy. These models describe therapist and client as team members collaborating on finding a solution, with language, rather than action, being the medium for change. All that's needed is a conversation, and reality will change as the therapist and client discuss the solutions they want to construct (Berg & de Shazer, 1993). In this sense, there's no hierarchy in solution-focused therapy. Collaborative approaches offer a refreshing focus on the therapist and client as a unit. Collaborative therapists take a closer look at what the client brings to the therapy while they themselves remain less central to the process. Clients who don't want to be directed feel a different sense of relationship with the therapist, one that's designed to raise their status by their sense of collaboration. Clients are viewed as the experts, and all solutions are seen as coming from them rather than from the therapist. Collaborative therapists believe that their clients feel a greater sense of ownership of their own solutions.

Solution-focused collaborative approaches direct their attention almost exclusively to the future (de Shazer, 1985). A primary concept of solution-focused therapy, maintaining a future focus, has been a powerful technique used by strategic therapists for 30 years. This emphasis on the future can be extremely helpful in focusing clients away from their present and past pain so they can see what's possible.

The strength of collaborative, nonauthoritarian approaches in emphasizing the client and minimizing the importance of the therapist is also one of these approaches' most troubling aspects. Fifty years have been spent demonstrating to therapists that they must learn specific skills they can offer clients. Brief therapy approaches have brought with them a view of therapy as a service profession in which clients ask for help and therapists must be able to offer answers. The field has moved toward the idea that therapists must know what to do in very serious situations. Nichols (1993) wrote:

If arranging and hosting conversations were all that a therapist did, that person should be called a mediator, or the opposite of a talk show host (whose aim is to arrange conversations that are nasty and abusive). The therapist as host neglects the role of teacher—a much maligned but essential aspect of any transformative therapy.

Proponents of conversational and solution-focused collaborative approaches believe that clients have the answers they need for creating change in their lives. There's some truth to this assertion. Certainly, the client offers information that shows the therapist which way to go to be helpful. In fact, in the approach to treatment described in this book, aggressive teenagers are viewed as providing the keys to reversing situations in which they're abusing their parents. In directive therapy, however, unlike solution-focused and other collaborative approaches, therapists are asked to use that information to devise strategies for change.

Aggressive adolescents teach us the nature of power and demonstrate how to use that power. Teenagers use the power of conspiracy and collusion to bring about outcomes that suit them. Therapists must help parents fight fire with fire by harnessing the power of conspiracy and collusion themselves and must help them design approaches that enable them to take charge of potentially dangerous situations.

Families in which teenagers are emotionally or physically abusing their parents have been the target population for the use of a unique strategy that's become known at the Michigan Family Institute as the "secret weapon strategy." Therapists must figure out how to keep control of the treatment of adolescents in the hands of their families. Keeping this control may not be possible once serious violent acts have been committed and laws broken, but it should be possible to maintain parental control of the therapy of adolescents who act *as if* they're going to be violent. These bad actors use gestures, facial expressions, words, and aggressive acts against objects or walls to convince parents and professionals that they're violent and dangerous. These dramatic teenagers act as if they're dangerous—and are responded to as if they are. In fact, many aggressive teenagers haven't committed a single harmful act against a person. Therefore, it would be an error to call a teenager violent when he or she hasn't harmed anyone.

CLINICAL VIGNETTE: A CLASSIC BAD ACTOR

Fourteen-year-old James and his younger brother were brought to therapy by his parents, Michael and Rose, who were in their mid-40s. These mild-mannered parents clearly abhorred violence. Michael was a large man who appeared unusually tired and worn for his age. Rose spoke in a kindly voice that belied her hidden anger. James, a blond, blue-eyed, muscular young man, was a B and C student who, according to reports from school, got along reasonably well with others and was respectful in class. James loved competitive wrestling, and Michael and Rose had always encouraged this interest.

The problem centered around the way James would quietly resist taking direction from his father. Whether Michael asked him to take out the garbage or do his homework, James would find a way to avoid doing what he requested. James would persist in his resistance until Michael screamed at him. Despite his father's anger, James still refused to follow directions. As the conflict between father and son increased, James's anger would slowly escalate into a blind rage, and he would punch his fists through the drywall and doors. James would scream, "One of these days I'm going to kill you," or "I'll kick your ass," and he'd raise his hand as if to hit his father. He would lapse into long tirades about how unfair his father was and could successfully stimulate guilty feelings in Michael about being too mean. After all, Rose had always accused her husband of being too hard on the children. James reinforced his image in his parents' eyes as a violent person by regularly telling them stories about some guys in school who were trying to start fights with him and how he planned to get a gun and set them straight once and for all. Yet the principal and teachers at James' school hadn't witnessed such violent scenes.

Michael and Rose became so frightened of their son's violent temper that they in turn threatened him—but they were afraid to apply real pressure. When they tried to impose consequences, James screamed, swore at them, and punched the walls (he had even hurt his knuckles punching a wall that was more solid than he'd anticipated). Previous therapists had reinforced the parents' fears by diagnosing James as suffering from "explosive personality disorder." After an apparently psychotic incident in which he was found angrily swinging his fists at the empty air, James was admitted to the adolescent unit of a local psychiatric hospital for treatment. Since he was believed to have had an acute psychotic episode, James was medicated with antipsychotic drugs; he was sent home after 3 weeks of treatment. His parents, however, still lived in fear of their son's temper. In fact, they were more frightened than before because his dangerousness was permanently recorded in a hospital record that labeled him with the diagnosis of acute schizophrenia, a condition the doctors said was likely to reemerge. James could now provide medical evidence that he was violent and unable to control his rage. But what had he actually done that was dangerous?

James was angry, confused, and unable to control himself. In order to keep him from being hospitalized again as a schizophrenic, it was imperative that his therapist intervene in the perceived "dangerousness" in the first two therapy sessions. The therapist knew that helping create observable change in the teen would be more successful than trying to convince parents and teachers that James wasn't really as troubled as he looked. Once James's behavior actually improved, his therapist reasoned, the boy could be seen as a more treatable case of misbehavior, a diagnosis both parents and professionals would be comfortable dealing with.

The presence of a cloud of doom was felt by James's parents and teachers; everyone had become confused and disoriented. No one seemed to know how to reason with this boy who was reacting so unreasonably. One unsuccessful response had already been attempted, namely, the overreaction of diagnosing adolescent rebellion as a medical problem and putting a sane boy in a psychiatric hospital. The following intervention offered a means by which James could be understood as a teenager who simply wanted his own way. The sinister cloud was destroyed as James's behavior improved. This intervention isn't intended for use with adolescents who've caused serious harm or carried out significant criminal acts. It's intended for use against aggression that could become serious violence, rather than against violence itself. Done well, the intervention reduces the chances of further hospitalization, other professional intervention, labeling, and medication.

DEFINING THE SECRET WEAPON STRATEGY

The secret weapon strategy, or a slight variation of it, has been attempted with about 50 cases in which the client would not have responded to straightforward contracting and directives. Despite our belief that the young people in these cases wouldn't have really hurt anyone, the families were nevertheless coached to have a plan by which a friend, neighbor, relative, or even a hired guard would be available to restrain any violent outburst that occurred. To date there has been only one case in which a client attacked another person.

The secret weapon strategy begins with the therapist joining the family's view of their child as a dangerous person. In the case of James, the therapist dramatized for Michael and Rose how their son's provocative and threatening behavior could lead to criminal acts or, if it occurred in the wrong place at the wrong time, could get James seriously hurt or killed. The therapist intentionally became more dramatic and pessimistic in order to escalate the parents' upset over James's threats and get them ready to take action. When Michael and Rose seemed sufficiently distressed and were talking with determination about the need to take action, the therapist asked them to agree that something must be done quickly. Timed properly, this kind of conversation usually ends with an agreement, because the parents have already acknowledged how urgent the situation is and how determined they are to stop it. The therapist asked Michael and Rose to take charge of James's acts and threats of aggression. In that session the parents generated a list of specific acts that they felt had to be stopped. The behaviors that therapists ask parents to list are often described as acts that are so dangerous that they must never happen again. These behaviors must be specific, and the therapist must keep parents from including behaviors that aren't dangerous, such as not doing homework or not mowing the lawn. James helped his parents and therapist make the list. Some examples are as follows:

- Threatening anyone's life
- Hitting plaster walls
- Breaking valuable objects
- Striking a sibling hard enough to cause marks or injury
- Staying out all night without anyone knowing his whereabouts
- Any criminal act
- Use of alcohol or drugs

Michael and Rose were then told to go out for an evening or afternoon in the next week without James and to decide during that time on something horrible they would do to their son the next time he committed an act of real or threatened aggression. Even if the act of aggression was not one associated with harm, if it appeared on the list, the devastation of the consequences was to compare to the parents' usual punishments the way an atom bomb compares to a firecracker.

The key to the secret weapon intervention is that the parents must agree with the therapist that the child cannot know what the secret weapon is. This shared secret put incredible power back in Michael and Rose's hands after months of feeling disenfranchised by both their children and by the system of professionals who had been dealing with him. James threatened to attack his brother in order to find out their secret. The therapist's task at that moment was to encourage them to stand firm and not be bullied by their son. Michael and Rose made the pact to impose the secret weapon if James were to do any of the acts on the list.

The secret weapon interventions chosen by parents have ranged from mildly horrible, to incredibly horrible depending on the seriousness of the offense. Some examples are as follows:

- Selling all stereo equipment and tapes belonging to their son or daughter
- Accompanying the teenager to school, sitting in class, and escorting him or her between classes

♦ Sending the child to live for a month with a friend or relative in another state who has a personality that comes as close as possible to that of a marine drill sergeant

♦ Pawning the child's possessions to pay for damages resulting from aggression or pay a fine (the pawnbroker technique in Chapter 6)

♦ Selling the child's designer clothing

♦ Removing all clothing belonging to the offender from the house, except what is currently being worn, for a fixed period of time

One set of parents wanted to show the teachers and principal of their son's school a videotape of a therapy session in which their son acted ridiculously and aggressively. This was a powerful intervention because the teachers thought the boy was an angel, and the boy himself seemed intent on their keeping this benevolent image of him. (This case history is described in Chapter 10.)

IMPLEMENTING THE SECRET WEAPON STRATEGY

In another case, 14-year-old Latasha had been sneaking out in the middle of the night and meeting boys. She was once found smoking pot in the yard at 2:00 A.M., and she often skipped school. Her parents didn't know where she was most of the time. They had tried everything—or so they thought—but to no avail. Working with a therapist, her parents concluded that if they could keep Latasha in school, they could demonstrate their ability to take charge of her. After working up a list of behaviors that could never be allowed to happen again, her parents decided on a secret weapon: The next time Latasha slipped out or skipped school, they would escort her to school and sit beside her in each class for a day. They were granted permission by the school principal to implement this plan, and they made sure that a few other relatives would be available if they needed to physically take Latasha to school. This wasn't a typical consequence for adolescent misbehavior—but, then, these weren't typical misbehaviors. What became of Latasha? Once she got the message that her parents meant what they said, Latasha became generally more compliant and began acting as if she needed her parents' permission before she did things. Once Latasha was back in school, her parents learned that she was having learning problems, and they were able to get her special help. Her parents never did have to escort her to school and keep her company in class.

Therapists may have to spend a great deal of time exploring what consequences each set of parents would be willing to carry out. It can be helpful for therapists to verbally walk parents through the experience of dealing with their child when he or she violates the sanction against destructive behavior. For instance, the therapist might ask parents to pretend that they have just awakened at 2:30 A.M. on a Sunday and have discovered that their child is nowhere to be found. The therapist can then ask the following questions: How would you implement the secret weapon without further threats, comments, or warnings? How could you see to it that the secret weapon just happens? Who would do what? How would you help each other avoid discussing your decision with your child?

If parents can be given a visual image of themselves carrying out the consequence they have agreed on, they're more likely to follow through if their child commits one of the acts on the list of dangerous acts they've drawn up. Young people who take a threatening stance without causing true harm to people and who predominantly make idle threats won't risk finding out what the secret weapon is—if the therapist has done a good job of setting the scene. A therapist can wait a week or two before implementing the strategy if parents seem reluctant. If parents aren't ready to proceed, it's perfectly fine to discuss their hesitancy; the therapist should make it clear that it will be up to the parents to decide when and if the strategy will be used. The pressure is on the parents more than the therapist; after all, they have to go home and live with their child for another week.

In the rare case of an adolescent who tests the limits once the parents have generated a list of specific behaviors the therapist can encourage the parents to carry out the agreed-upon consequence and to then think of a more severe secret weapon; their child obviously didn't feel frightened enough by the milder secret weapon as a deterrent. This was the case with 17-year-old Marnie, who was screaming and yelling at home, had begun to shove her mother around, and had recently pushed her mother to the floor. Her parents loved her so dearly they couldn't quite grasp the idea of doing something painful. Out of sympathy for their pain, I allowed them to choose a secret weapon consequence that was really too weak, namely, taking away Marnie's stereo and all of her CDs. The parents were uncomfortable with the idea of selling Marnie's stereo equipment. I knew that Marnie's parents weren't ready to take charge, but I went along with their plan because I felt a combination of sympathy for them and fear of driving them out of therapy by pushing too hard. Marnie, who sensed that there were no teeth behind her parents' threats, violated her guidelines the next day. Her parents might have dropped out of therapy after such a precipitous failure. Fortunately, they became more angry and determined. They imposed the penalty they'd chosen, and readily agreed to a more severe secret weapon. They decided that if there were further violations they would to put all Marnie's belongings in storage, except those she needed to survive. Marnie sensed that they meant business and stopped all of the assaultive behavior that had previously become a daily occurrence.

If the therapist anticipates that an adolescent will react to the secret weapon strategy by retaliating in a way that could endanger someone, the therapist must spend more time with the parents designing a strategy that will ensure everyone's safety. Does the father feel comfortable that he can safely restrain his son? Should younger children be in the house with their brother without a parent? Does the mother feel comfortable that she can restrain her daughter, or should her husband be home whenever she is? Should arrangements be made with a friend or family member to be readily available or even to move in for a while so that another adult is always there to help restrain the adolescent? If their child were to run away, what would the parents' plan be for getting him or her back quickly?

It should be noted that one parent is rarely able to be convincing enough to stop a teenager from violating the mandate to stop all violent behaviors. The child often knows that the parent doesn't have enough resolve to follow through with a painful consequence. Thus, a single parent would do well to find a relative who can participate in therapy sessions; the two would constitute a coparenting dyad that an adolescent would find more unpredictable than his or her mother or father alone.

Adolescents properly treated with the secret weapon strategy rarely violate the guidelines provided by their parents. Therefore, they never learn what their parents' secret weapon was going to be. I often jokingly suggest to parents that they give their child a letter revealing the nature of the secret weapon as a wedding or college graduation gift. Parents find humor in their child's predicament, which brings the parents closer to each other. Once set in motion, the secret weapon strategy changes the case status from "critical" to "typical."

After a child's behavior improves, parents often say that he or she appeared possessed by demons and that now the child they knew and loved is back. Through use of the secret weapon strategy, the natural hierarchy of the family is restored; parents are in charge, and children acknowledge their parents' authority. However, the therapy of a troubled family remains to be completed, for there's often a reason for the emergence of such dangerous behavior. A major step has been taken, though and the case is now treatable. The sinister cloud has dissipated, and parents who were in terrible conflict over their child have begun to feel unified and empowered. By the way, I suspect these changes in the parents and in the family structure were what the aggressive adolescent was trying to accomplish by behaving so badly in the first place.

NINE

He Must Be on Drugs

How does the suspicion that an adolescent may be using drugs or alcohol complicate a therapist's ability to think clearly and devise a plan? Would that sinister cloud be harder to banish than adolescent aggression alone? What if the teenager *is* using drugs? How different would the treatment be? What if an adolescent isn't using drugs or alcohol but everyone thinks he or she is? These questions and many others about the relationship between adolescent aggression and substance abuse are addressed in the following pages. First, consider the following scenario:

You are invited to a high school staffing meeting for a student you're treating in therapy. Your 15-year-old client, Mary, is skipping classes and screaming at teachers, and her grades have dropped from A's and B's, to C's and D's. Having met with the family, you have a lot of ideas about why such a competent young woman would become troubled and defy her parents and teachers. After introductions are made, each person at the table has a chance to comment on his or her impressions of why Mary's performance and behavior have deteriorated over the last 6 months.

Having sat in on many school staffings, you spend the time driving to the school rehearsing what you'll say in response to the one comment you know will inevitably be made. With a knowing look, someone in the room will say, "Maybe she's on drugs." There will be a pregnant pause as the members of the staffing silently decide whether or not to follow up this comment by discontinuing the discussion on the possible sources of Mary's problems and recommending that she be referred to a program specializing in drug treatment for an assessment. Your sole function at the meeting may be to block this derailment of the process and keep everyone on track by stating that you consider drugs to be an inadequate explanation for Mary's behavior. Then you can encourage everyone to think creatively about what conditions in Mary's life could cause such a change for the worse.

The hard part of your job will be to convince everyone in the room that even if Mary is smoking pot, drugs aren't necessarily the real problem. Bad choices, a need for more parental involvement, a need for more structure in the school setting, serious family problems that are hurting the people Mary loves—these are more likely to be the causes of the deterioration in her behavior. People too quickly assume that a student who isn't doing well in school must be on drugs—*and* that drugs are the root of all of his or her problems. Marijuana use doesn't necessarily explain why a teen's grades are slipping or why he or she is getting into fights. Accepting drug use as a universal explanation for adolescent problems is a mistake.

CAPTURING THE DEMON

The assumption that drugs are the culprit is a problem because such a leap of logic takes the spotlight off everyone's responsibility to find new, creative solutions for an adolescent's problems. There was a time when acting-out teenagers were thought to be possessed by demons and therefore unable to control their own behavior. Parents were exonerated of responsibility for correcting their child's behavior because the problem was considered a spiritual issue that parents have no control over.

Just as it was once commonly believed that demons could move from person to person and were beyond the influence of mere mortals, there is now a common misunderstanding that when young people use LSD they immediately lead their friends to use it as well and that drug use is something about which parents can do little. The stereotypical scenario of a drug-using teenager begins with an image of a good boy who had few problems and whose life was going well. Then, the story goes, someone introduced him to marijuana and the drug, like a demon, took control of him. His grades began to drop, he began hanging around with kids who were a bad influence, and he acted angry all the time.

Just as parents of mentally ill teens are told that the disease is the sole problem, the parents of teens who use drugs are also told that they can't do anything to help except refer their son or daughter to a specialized treatment program.

ASSESSING THE PROBLEM

When 14-year-old Mark began getting into fights, no one was sure what had come over him. He skipped school and was seen hanging around with a group of boys who were known to be troublemakers. Mark's school counselor automatically assumed that the boy was on drugs, but after talking to Mark and his parents, she learned that Mark's grandmother had died recently and that the entire family had become depressed. Although many children do experiment with marijuana and other drugs, there are usually more direct explanations for poor grades or misbehavior.

Twelve-year-old Maria started spending most of her time in her room. Her parents were no longer sure where she was when Maria went out. Because Maria was avoiding them, her parents began to wonder whether she was using drugs and isolating herself to keep them from detecting signs of drug use in her. As it turned out, Maria had just begun junior high school and was having trouble adjusting to more difficult classes and an increased workload. What she was avoiding was her homework.

Sixteen-year-old Frank found himself in an awkward position when his father came home unexpectedly and caught him smoking marijuana. Frank's father jumped to the conclusion that marijuana use explained why Frank had become more moody and disrespectful in the past month. When the family came to me for therapy, a very different story unfolded. Usually a compliant boy, Frank was having more and more trouble accepting his father's overprotectiveness; his father was having trouble making the transition to negotiating with his son rather than laying down the law. A few sessions spent discussing with Frank's father how to negotiate and where to draw the line as a parent solved the problem.

CLINICAL VIGNETTE: THE DRUGGIE

The following transcript is a good example of how parents who accept the idea that the presence of drugs explains their child's misbehavior fail to look any further for explanations. The Parsons family lived in a small rural town and commuted to our program in another rural town to avoid being seen going into a mental health clinic.

Derek was 15 years old and seemed like a clean-cut fellow. His brown hair was cut neatly, and his yellow shirt and new jeans were fashionable. Mr. Parsons, an overweight man in his 40s, wore a sport coat and jeans. Mrs. Parsons had ginger-colored hair, was dressed in a business suit, and had a generally business-like manner. Mr. and Mrs. Parsons sat next to each other, with their legs crossed toward each other. Derek sat next to Mr. Parsons, and his 11-year-old brother, Frank, who sat quietly looking down, was seated next to Mrs. Parsons. This symmetry suggested a healthy, well-balanced family.

I began by asking, "What are the concerns that bring you here today?"

Mrs. Parsons began describing their situation. "Derek was admitted . . . was assessed for . . . let me start again. Derek was admitted to Westchester to be assessed for some kind of treatment for chemical abuse. He was accepted into the program. When Derek went into the program—" She stopped suddenly and turned to Derek, asking, "Is this okay if I talk about this in front of your brother?"

Derek responded, "I don't care."

Mrs. Parsons continued, "Okay. When Derek went into Westchester, he took drugs with him. So he never was really free of drugs for the week. He would never go back there again. He's agreed to counseling because, certainly, we know that we need professional help. It's not something Michael, Frank, myself, even Derek can do. Derek has said he's trying to go straight. I have some doubt about that."

This presentation was typical of a parent attempting to deal with a child on drugs. Mrs. Parsons's statement that there wasn't anything any family member could do in the face of drugs shows the kind of helplessness parents feel. Mr. and Mrs. Parsons had turned to the experts for help, but Derek had defeated the treatment program from the start. I began presenting the idea that Derek's drug use was an issue of willpower rather than of disease or genetics. I ignored comments of helplessness and only responded to those that addressed whether or not Derek was really trying to quit.

"Trying and succeeding may be two different things," I said.

When I made a critical comment, Mrs. Parsons became more positive. Her response to my negativity suggested to me that she said critical things only with great effort and tended to assume a protective role. "He might be trying," Mrs. Parsons said. "I don't see him as despondent as he was before he went into Westchester. He seems to be a nicer kid since he came home. It's great to have him home. We really missed him."

Moving back to information gathering, I asked, "What kind of drugs did Derek get involved in?"

"Derek can tell you about that in confidentiality. I don't want Frank to hear about that," Mrs. Parsons said.

"That's something I need to know, so maybe we'll have to excuse Frank for a few minutes since you folks need to hear it also."

"We already know," she said.

I concluded, "Frank, I hate to put you out there by yourself, but parents make decisions about what they want their kids to hear and what they don't. I'll get back to you as quick as we can, okay?" Frank allowed me to lead him to the door without comment and went to the waiting room. Mrs. Parsons was trying to exclude herself and her husband from the interview, so I had to find a way to keep them in. They'd been taught that there was nothing they could do about Derek's drug problem. If I'd let them leave the office, too, I would have given them the impression that I was going to solve the problem alone.

I began asking about Derek's drug use because a basic clinical issue had to be settled early in therapy. A therapist must figure out whether a teenage client is addicted to drugs or alcohol before deciding how to proceed. My experience has been that very few adolescents coming into therapy are addicted to the point where they can't stop using drugs. Physiological withdrawal symptoms are rare. True addicts are more likely to downplay their drug use and to act as if there's no reason for concern. Addicted adolescents rarely admit to drug use. Nonaddicted teens who use drugs can be viewed as children who are experiencing and drawing attention to family problems. These symptomatic teens often brag about their misbehavior and flaunt their drug or alcohol use in front of their parents. As was the case with Derek, symptomatic teens freely describe their drug use and even embellish their accounts of how much they use and how often. That symptomatic teens dramatize their drug use makes sense. If a teenager's reason for using drugs is to draw as much attention as possible to a troubled situation, that teen would make sure as many adults as possible knew about his or her drug use. Symptomatic teens usually go out of their way to come home or show up at school under the influence of drugs or alcohol.

Derek's mother approached him as if he were an addict who'd therefore be reluctant to speak about his addiction, but Derek turned out to be a symptomatic boy who described his drug use in an almost jaunty tone. Had he been an addict, he wouldn't have freely offered details about the extent of his drug and alcohol use. In general, a therapist should multiply an addict's report of drug use by three; the symptomatic child's report of drug use should be divided by at least three.

Mrs. Parsons began, "This is completely up to you, Derek."

"I know. I've admitted I used drugs," he answered.

"What drugs were you using when you were admitted to Westchester?" I asked.

"Pot."

"Mainly marijuana? Anything else?"

"Sometimes coke."

"With any regularity? Daily? Weekly? Monthly?"

"Maybe monthly. I don't know."

I was pretty sure Derek was symptomatic rather than addicted, so I chose to play down his reference to cocaine rather than let him frighten his parents by emphasizing one of the most addictive drugs in existence. I knew I could always discuss cocaine use with him alone at another time to make sure I wasn't overlooking anything. I responded, "So you were more experimenting with that one."

"Uh-huh."

"How about the pot use?"

"Daily."

"A joint a day? Two joints? Three?"

"About a joint a day."

"What was your time of day? Morning? During school? After school? Evening?"

"Usually after I got home from school. I don't smoke pot in school. I didn't go to school the whole last quarter."

I asked, "How did that come about?"

For the first time Mr. Parsons offered an explanation. "He left for school in the morning—"

Before he could continue, Derek cut in, commenting, "I lost credit, and then I didn't see much sense in going back."

I tried to get a feel for whether Derek's parents were paying close enough attention to Derek's whereabouts so that the same mistake wouldn't happen again. I asked, "How long was Derek skipping before you found out, and how did you find out?"

Mrs. Parsons began again as the narrator, but Mr. Parsons was becoming more involved in the discussion. "Well, we started getting the absentee slips from school. Each class sent one, and by the time we put that all together, he wasn't even going to school."

Mr. Parsons agreed: "It took several weeks."

I've always assumed that if you criticize people, especially in the first session, they'll get even with you. Getting even usually takes the form of withholding information or not following directives, so I softened the implied criticism by saying, "They sure took their time about letting you know, didn't they?"

"Yes, they did," Mrs. Parsons quickly agreed, sounding a bit relieved.

I wanted to change the subject to avoid leaving these parents feeling criticized and uncooperative, so I went back to exploring their treatment history and attempting to determine what preconceptions they may have had about teenagers and drugs. I asked, "Westchester's program usually includes a lot of family involvement. Were you involved in any family sessions while Derek was there?"

Mrs. Parsons said, "Uh-huh."

"What did you think of that part of the program? Treatment programs work differently, and it would help me to understand what you learned in that process."

Mr. Parsons offered, "We only were there for one day, Friday. He ran away from the program the next Friday, and that would have been the first day the kids would have been with the adults. That session never happened, so we held it in our own house when he wouldn't go back. It was left at the point where his behavior pattern was in a lot more trouble than we thought. The session we went to helped us see that his use of drugs, using more and more of it, apparently caused everything to start to deteriorate. School, activities, his trouble with the police, his trouble obeying the rules. Finally, one time, his behavior was just becoming intolerable. At that point we took him to Westchester with the idea that he either had to get help or he would have to leave. If he wants to move out with his buddies and do that, fine, but not in our house."

As is often the case in families, the apparently quiet parent was the one who had a very strong position. Mr. Parsons's opinion, once spoken, was stronger than his wife's, which was expressed in a more placating tone. Mr. Parsons's definitive position smacked of an ultimatum. Rather than point out the obvious difference between the parents' styles, I continued to solicit information that would help me assess the seriousness of Derek's drug involvement. "When did you first become aware of things with Derek that concerned you?"

Mrs. Parsons answered, "This school year. Especially the last 5 months."

Mr. Parsons added, "Last marking period he was doing fine. And then, just everything went."

Wandering slightly off the subject, Derek said, "Once I lost credit, I didn't see any point."

His father added, "But we worked it out with the school that he would get credit if he went through Westchester. But he wouldn't go back."

Derek had suddenly revived the subject of school attendance and credit loss, and his father had opposed him on it. Then his mother tried to direct the discussion back to the topic of their previous therapy. Derek seemed to be showing me that his going back to school was a significant area of controversy for his parents. I then explored Mr. and Mrs. Parsons's ability to agree by asking, "How would you know when things are getting better?"

True to my assumption that he was the more forceful parent, Mr. Parsons immediately answered, "Derek will go back to school and save his grades for the year. If he can't, he can go to summer school. He says he wants to continue school next fall. He'll do his share of the work around the house."

Mrs. Parsons answered in a meeker tone, saying, "It would be nice if I didn't have to worry every time the phone rings at work. Every time someone told me it was Michael on the phone, my heart would sink."

Mrs. Parsons's reference to her heart sinking when her husband called was made in the context of his delivering bad news about Derek's behavior, but her statement could also have been a metaphorical message about her general feelings toward her husband. Derek's blatant use of marijuana and other drugs was looking more and more to me like an attempt to direct his parents away from a serious problem between them. Rather than being a drug addict, Derek appeared to be a young man who craved reassurance that his parents still cared about him and who was concerned about what the tension between his parents meant.

It's important to offer people hope for improvement from the very beginning of therapy. I began forming a hypothesis that Derek's symptoms were embedded in a struggle between his parents. I needed to find out the nature of that struggle but knew that it was important for Mr. and Mrs. Parsons to be aware of my good opinion of them, an awareness that would help me elicit further information about their conflicts in later discussions. I concluded that part of the session by saying, "So you would need to see a change that continued for a while so that you could get your trust back. I see you both still have a lot of positive feelings for Derek."

Mrs. Parsons said, "Yeah, we love him."

Mr. Parsons said, "We wouldn't be here if we didn't."

"That's great," I said, adding, "And it increases the chances that this problem's going to get solved quickly and completely."

Derek's parents were having trouble agreeing about how to intervene with their son, and that conflict was undoubtedly being fueled by other disagreements they were having. At this point I felt it best to end on a note of agreement between the parents in order to begin a pattern of more cooperation in dealing with their son.

AVAILABLE OPTIONS FOR DRUG TREATMENT

If a therapist concludes that he or she is dealing with a drug-abusing adolescent who may be addicted, it's critical that assistance be obtained from a drug treatment center that has medical facilities. Many people can be detoxified and withdrawn from drugs on an outpatient basis. In some cases an inpatient program may be needed; this decision should be based on the level of abuse or addiction or because of the failure of an outpatient detox attempt.

Detox and treatment done at home and supervised by the family have some logical advantages. Often, one or both parents of a drug-abusing teen are also abusing drugs or alcohol. Traditional theory suggests that this fact makes treatment difficult or impossible. In-home treatment allows the therapist to impose the same limitations, such as abstinence, as those required of the young drug abuser on other family members. The house must be emptied of all alcohol and other addictive substances, which often makes it harder for other abusers in the house to continue.

Parents with addictive problems must go through the process with their child as he or she withdraws, struggles, relapses, and succeeds. What parents must say to their child to help him or her through detox and treatment at home is often what they need to be saying to themselves and to each other. Therefore, the in-home treatment process is therapeutic in many ways; it does more than address the individual struggle of an adolescent.

Many issues have to be considered while deciding when and how to get an adolescent off drugs. If a teenager isn't addicted, it's best to avoid inpatient programs and the risk that the program will become the expert instead of the parents. If medical detox is needed, it's possible to arrange an outpatient detoxification with a physician or psychiatrist. Use of intensive outpatient and traditional inpatient treatment programs are alternatives to family-focused outpatient treatment rather than adjuncts. Most traditional programs, including self-help programs, give advice, direct change, define the problem, and generally act like therapists.

Once an addicted adolescent is drug-free, the therapy becomes like any other family therapy. Drug use can then be treated like any other symptom that parents must learn to take charge of. If the underlying problem is related to other family conflicts, as it was with the Parsons family, therapy addresses those problems in addition to helping parents take control of their child's drug use.

GETTING AT THE PROBLEM

The End of Session 1

As the first session with the Parsons family was wrapping up, I didn't have a good theory about why Derek was using drugs and skipping school. When it's the end of a session and I don't have a clear plan, I fall back on Rule 1 for directive therapists: When in doubt as to what to direct clients to do, advise them to take a reasonable step back toward normality, in order to see how they handle the task. Such a step often reveals necessary information.

In Derek's case the most straightforward strategy was to convince his parents to send him back to school. Despite loss of credit, students are never harmed by sitting in their classes and learning. Mr. and Mrs. Parsons and I planned how they would get Derek to school and how he would get home. I felt that if the parents could work together to get Derek to school, their success might indicate that the conflicts between them weren't too severe. On the other hand, if their differences interfered with a task as simple as getting their son to school, I could assume more serious difficulties between them.

Session 2

Mr. and Mrs. Parsons walked into Session 2 with Derek in tow. He sat between them with a different, more serious, expression on his face. I asked how Derek did in school, without directing the question to anyone in particular, and was surprised when Mr. Parsons spoke first. He said, "He didn't go to school." When I asked why he didn't go to school, Mr. Parsons again answered, "Two of us thought he shouldn't go, and I'm not even going to get into that." The face-off had begun between mother and father. At that point in the therapy I asked myself the question, "Do they just disagree about Derek or have we got a bigger problem within the marriage?"

Sessions 3 and 4: Moving in Unison

Taking the path I felt Mr. and Mrs. Parsons were most likely to accept, I worked on getting them to agree on decisions about Derek and on acting in unison. Over the next two sessions I challenged them to come together and predicted that Derek might do something to stop them from taking charge of him. I decided that if Derek accepted his parents' united authority, I would proceed as if their disagreements were only about him. On the other hand, if Derek acted worse in the face of his parents' unity, I would take the misbehavior as his way of saying that he had no faith in this show of parental cooperation and that he knew it was a sham. Derek would have a way of telling me that he was aware of greater problems between his parents.

Derek was arrested between the third and fourth family therapy sessions for breaking into garages and stealing tools. My hypothesis that there were more serious problems between his parents was confirmed. We spent two sessions negotiating consequences for Derek's crime and discussing how he would make restitution and to what extent his parents would agree to try to get him off the hook for his actions. Derek's parents began applying new pressure on him by agreeing on the consequences for his crime.

As his parents became more unified in dealing with him, Derek arranged for them to find a bag of marijuana in his room and a pot pipe constructed from aluminum foil. The marijuana was a powerful invitation to again explain Derek's criminal behavior as the result of drug use. However, if I'd accepted this detour, Mr. and Mrs. Parsons would have given up their restitution plan and all the structure we'd worked out and would once again have seen the solution to Derek's problem as beyond their abilities. To help Mr. and Mrs. Parsons stick to the subject of parental authority, I examined the pot pipe they'd brought with them, looked at Derek, and said, "This is really a miserable excuse for a pipe. Couldn't you do any better than this?" Because I wasn't terrified by the marijuana and the pipe, I was able to help Derek's parents make a calm decision to watch their son's comings and goings more closely to block access to such things. I then changed the topic back to restitution, return to school, and consequences, continuing as if we hadn't been interrupted.

Session 5 and Onward: The Revelation

In subsequent sessions I continued unifying Derek's parents and blocked their tendency to become helpless when their son did things that frightened them. When looking for information, a discussion about the future often surfaces a great deal. For example, when Mr. Parsons's turn arrived in a discussion we were having about each family member's plans for the future, Derek mumbled, "And you're going to Texas." I had to ask Derek to repeat what he'd said, but before he could do so, his parents launched into an explanation of Mr. Parsons's plans to take a job in Texas. He was intending to leave in 6 weeks. When I asked Mr. and Mrs. Parsons more about the plans to move, it became clear that they hadn't discussed this very much. I then asked whether the move was a job opportunity or a separation. Mr. Parsons said it was a job opportunity, and Mrs. Parsons said she felt her husband was leaving her for an old girlfriend in Texas. She hadn't agreed to this plan. In fact, Mr. and Mrs. Parsons hadn't agreed about when and if he'd return or if she would move to Texas to join him.

The move was discussed over the course of the next three sessions, and Mr. Parsons reassured his wife that he had no intention of leaving her. They agreed on when the family would visit Mr. Parsons in Texas and also on how long he would work to establish himself professionally there. They agreed that if Mr. Parsons was not successful in an agreed-upon period of time, he'd move back home; on the other hand, if he was successful enough to allow Mrs. Parsons to leave her job, she and the children would move to Texas to join him.

Until Mr. Parsons left for Texas, we met for sessions regularly and discussed how Mrs. Parsons would be handling the children during his absence. Knowing that she had to get ready to do the job by herself, she became more forceful over the course of these weeks, talked tougher, and imposed more serious consequences for the children's misbehavior. Derek went back to school and maintained reasonably good grades. He no longer skipped classes, and there weren't any further reports of drugs. Once Derek saw that his parents stayed in touch after his father's move and that he still had a dad, he continued to settle down. A few sessions after Mr. Parsons left for Texas, Mrs. Parsons reported that things were going well, and she ended the therapy.

At a 1-year follow-up, Derek was still in the same school, was attending regularly, and his grades were B's and C's. Mr. Parsons was still in Texas, and he and Mrs. Parsons were moving toward a decision about whether the family would move to Texas or whether Mr. Parsons would come home.

If the standard assumption about adolescents being "taken over" by drugs had been applied to Derek, he might have adopted a lifelong identity as an addict. He might never have felt normal again and might have gone through a great deal of inpatient treatment in rehab centers. In all likelihood Derek would have grown progressively more troubled.

THE FACTS

Parents experience a generalized fear of alcohol and drugs and their effects on adolescents. Some solid information on adolescent drug use could help them develop a more balanced view of the demon. The following information may help a therapist properly inform parents. Before we proceed with this information, though, two points must be addressed.

First, we all know that alcohol and drug use among teenagers is common. Experimentation is common. But it isn't commonly known that most adolescents handle their drug and alcohol use without getting out of control. Second, I must concede that there are kids whose drug use is out of control. But as you read the statistics in the following paragraphs, please ask yourself whether the drug use of your adolescent clients is addiction or whether they, like Derek, are reacting to something else. Any reader will agree that serious drug users need to change their behavior. But ask yourself this question: "Is addiction such a powerful force that the usual principles of behavior change don't apply?" I assume the usual principles of behavior change remain the same whether a particular teenager's problem is drugs, alcohol, sexual abuse, schizophrenia, or simple misbehavior.

In the following pages you'll read about the prevalence of alcohol and drug use among teenagers and will notice the relatively small percentages of adolescents using substances at high doses and high frequencies. However, the prevalence of drug and alcohol use indicated here is sufficient to support the idea that parents must know enough about alcohol and drugs to see the problem clearly rather than assume that their child is being "taken over."

A popular textbook reports that one-third of adolescents ages 12 to 17 reported using marijuana and that more than half of those used it in the 30 days preceding the study. Of that group 10% had used inhalants and hallucinogens, 7% had used alcohol, and 50% had smoked tobacco (Lawson & Lawson, 1992).

The NIDA Study

In another, larger survey the National Institute on Drug Abuse (NIDA; 1991) looked at current trends in alcohol and drug use by high school seniors. After alcohol and marijuana, the most commonly used illicit drugs were stimulants and inhalants. Hallucinogens were reported next in frequency of use, followed by (in descending order of frequency) cocaine, opiates other than heroin, sedatives, and tranquilizers. The information on types of drugs in the following paragraphs is from the same NIDA report.

Of particular concern to parents is cocaine. Cocaine comes in two forms: a white powder that's inhaled through the nose and "crack," which comes in small chunks or "rocks" that are smoked for a rapid, intense high. Among high school seniors 3.5% had tried crack; 1.9% had used it in the last year, and 0.7% had used it in the last month; 5.3% had used some form of cocaine, and 36% of those used crack. These are statistics for having tried cocaine, not for regular use or addiction. These are lower figures than I would have anticipated when considering the level of fear parents feel about their children becoming addicted to cocaine.

The inhalants most commonly used were amyl and butyl nitrites. These are legal drugs (used for heart stimulation) that produce a rapid increase in blood pressure, which creates a high. Street names are "poppers," "snappers," "locker room," and "rush." These inhalants had been tried by 1 in 50 students in this study.

PCP and LSD were the most prevalent hallucinogens used by the subjects. These drugs produce mood distortions and sensory illusions. PCP, a white powder, was used by 2.8% of seniors. LSD, known as "acid," was more heavily used, at 8.7%.

The opiates used by the subjects were, typically, prescription pain-killers containing codeine and Demerol, with 1 in 12 seniors reportedly using these opiates. Although 1.3% of the students admitted to ever using heroin, that was considered a low estimate.

The sedatives reportedly used include prescription barbiturates and the sedative-hypnotic methaqualone, or Quaaludes (or "Ludes"). Barbiturates were reportedly used by 6.8% of seniors and Quaaludes by 2.3%.

Prescription sedatives such as Valium, Librium, and Xanax, which are growing rapidly as drugs of abuse, weren't included in this study.

Nearly all students (90%) admitted to trying alcohol, with 57% being current users and 32% admitting to five or more drinks on at least one occasion in the last 2 weeks. Sixty-four percent had tried cigarettes, and 29% had smoked in the last month. These data indicate that alcohol is the drug parents should watch for most carefully.

Daily use of drugs was reported at a surprisingly low rate. Marijuana was used daily by 2.2% of seniors, alcohol by 3.7%, and other illicit drugs by less than 1%. Again, these statistics justify cause for serious concern, but they hardly suggest a demon waiting to pounce on our children. Parents have a tough job helping their drug- and alcohol-abusing children—but that job can be accomplished successfully.

SUBSTANCE ABUSE: COMPLICATION OR CAUSE OF PROBLEMS?

Parents are often told to look for very general symptoms to assess whether their child is using drugs. Mood swings and a drop in grades are considered warning signs. Although these symptoms may be signs of an alcohol or drug problem, they're also symptoms that typically accompany any of the following emotional traumas: the death of a family member, being jilted, the occurrence of domestic violence or sexual abuse, or the onset of depression in a parent or sibling. Parents should react strongly to a child's moodiness or drop in grades because these symptoms clearly indicate a serious problem—but not necessarily abuse of alcohol or drugs. They should vigorously pursue the cause of their child's symptoms while keeping an open mind about what the underlying problem might be. The parents' mission is to accurately identify the problem by digging deeply into the life of their child, who may be extremely talented at concealing any personal problem, including substance use.

To differentiate between substance abuse and other problems, it's wise for the therapist to direct parents to search for further signs of drug and alcohol use, such as intoxication, the smell of alcohol or marijuana, and the adolescent's sudden association with students who are known by the school and community to be drug involved. New friends who are poor students aren't necessarily drug users; an adolescent's association with them may reflect his or her own failure in school. The search for further signs of the presence of alcohol or drugs is always useful because the quest will either confirm or deny the presence of substance abuse, and it will often unearth the other problems that are the teenager's true concerns.

The conclusion that alcohol and drug use is a complication rather than a cause is supported by the U.S. Department of Health and Human Services (1993) in its publication *Guidelines for the Treatment of Alcohol and Other Drug Abusing Adolescents*. The authors were interested in adolescents involved in the juvenile justice system and wrote, "Most youths in the juvenile justice system abuse alcohol or other drugs (AOD's). This AOD abuse exacerbates other problems in their lives and makes any effort to rehabilitate them more difficult." The report suggests that the more a youth is involved with drugs, the more likely it is that he or she has a history of problems related to psychological disturbance or physical and sexual abuse. In fact, 70 to 95% of juveniles in detention have used alcohol or other drugs. In a study of juveniles admitted to a Colorado detention center 90% of girls and 58% of boys had been sexually abused. Of the sexually abused children, 70% reported anxiety and depression, 50% reported suicidal thoughts, and 25% had attempted suicide. It isn't a huge leap of logic to conclude that these problems contributed to substance abuse rather than the other way around.

A therapist or parent might assume that marijuana (read "the Devil") made a fellow like Derek Parsons start misbehaving and skipping school. But perhaps it makes more sense to understand that Derek was in emotional pain. He used drugs to ease the pain and to draw attention to his need for answers about his and his family's future. When a teenager uses alcohol and drugs, the therapist has a choice between seeing the substance use as the problem or as the result of a problem. The therapist must also choose whether to jump to the conclusion that alcohol or drugs are causing the adolescent's symptoms. Although the use of alcohol and drugs offers a quick and easy explanation for an adolescent's problems, that explanation is often simplistic and creates a smoke screen behind which the real concerns are hiding.

Aggression itself can be a smoke screen behind which other problems hide. In Chapter 10, I present the story of a boy who repeatedly threatened to murder his family and assorted therapists. He created an aura about himself of criminality despite not having actually hurt anyone. This boy's determination to draw attention to his potential for deadly aggression raised many questions about why a boy who hadn't been a problem before would suddenly become obsessed with hatred and murder.

TEN

The Clown

The Therapy of a 13-Year-Old Boy Threatening Murder

Early in my practice with adolescents I began to recognize the need for a method that could transform misused power into either respect or cooperative use of that power. The interview presented in the following transcript dates from the point at which I began a formal approach to the treatment of teenagers who threaten violence. The details of the process for carrying out the secret weapon strategy are discussed in Chapter 8. In addition to focusing on the secret weapon strategy and on ways to stop the violence, this transcript also shows the reader how to design interventions that address and resolve the reasons for aggression. Intervening in the family system requires the ability to move rapidly to stop aggression and violence as well as an understanding of why symptoms exist.

CLINICAL VIGNETTE

Mike was a 12-year-old in an inpatient program when I met him. Redheaded, tall and gangly, he didn't look at all threatening. His family lived in urban North Carolina and besides his mother and father included an 11-year-old sister, Bonnie, and a 16-year-old brother, Jim. Mike's mother, a schoolteacher with a master's degree, was becoming progressively more handicapped by multiple sclerosis; at that time, however, she was only moderately incapacitated. Mike's father was the manager for a furniture distributing firm.

The family's first consultation was with another therapist during a family meeting in the psychiatric hospital. At that time Mike's parents were upset because he'd been hospitalized after repeatedly breaking things at home and threatening to kill his family (he had threatened the lives of inpatient staff members as well). The inpatient therapist referred the case to me because his position would not allow him to provide outpatient treatment after Mike's release.

I met for my first session with Mr. and Mrs. Murphy the day before Mike was released from the hospital. Mrs. Murphy was tearful during much of the session because of her son's hospitalization. Her fragile appearance was similar to Mike's, and she appeared quite sad. She mentioned that her mother and father had both died within the last 3 years and that her mother-in-law had died during that time as well. Both parents agreed that the grandparents would have been appalled at Mike's confinement in a psychiatric hospital. In tears, Mrs. Murphy said that with the hospitalization it was as if Mike, too, were dead. Although it sounded like Mike had injured many people, a detailed history clarified that he hadn't done any actual physical harm to anyone—except for fights with his brother and sister, which, although rough, hadn't resulted in injury to them. I also learned that his 16-year-old brother, Jim, regularly physically disciplined Mike, using his skills as a judo expert, when he got out of control. Jim threw and pinned Mike to the ground whenever he thought Mike needed it.

Both parents sounded devastated while relating the tale of Mike's hospitalization. They'd been to a series of therapists, psychiatrists, and psychologists who specialized in treating adolescents, and each one had said that Mike was untreatable because he wouldn't talk to them about his feelings. Mike's parents begged him to speak to the professionals so that he could stay at home, but when he steadfastly refused to speak, Mr. and Mrs. Murphy finally gave in to the will of the experts and accepted that Mike was dangerous and untreatable and needed hospitalization. I encouraged Mr. and Mrs. Murphy to see themselves as the only ones who could help Mike. After I explained the philosophy of short-term change-oriented family therapy, they became interested. I helped them set guidelines Mike had to agree to abide by before they would allow him to return home, and they agreed to bring him home once he'd consented to these rules in writing. When his parents went to the hospital with their list of rules, Mike promptly demonstrated his willingness to abide by them and was released from the hospital the next day.

Session 1: Getting Off on the Right Foot

In my first session with Mike, both his parents were present. Mike refused to talk in their presence, but I explained that his silence wouldn't interfere with effective therapy. In the first part of the transcript, I'm talking with Mike alone after spending time just with his parents in order to gather information. I met with Mike in hopes of finding some common ground and getting him to agree to participate in the therapy. His parents sat anxiously in the waiting room during this interview, no doubt fearing that I was one more expert who would dash their hopes of Mike's ever having a normal life.

I began the interview with Mike by saying, "You know, Mike, my experience with guys who've been having the kinds of problems you have is that they're really worried. They worry about people they love who aren't doing so well—like your mother. You know, your mom's been really upset because of the deaths of her parents. She's got a physical illness that's getting worse and worse."

Grinning, Mike answered, "That means she can't make me do anything I don't want to do."

"You like that, huh?"

"I threatened to hit my younger sister. My parents said I threatened to hit my brother with a wrench, and I would have."

I was already beginning to wonder whether Mike was as dangerous as everyone thought, so I asked, "Have you ever done that?"

Mike continued as if he hadn't heard me. "I threatened to hit my brother with a baseball bat, and I almost did."

"You're good at almosts," I challenged. "You still haven't decided whether you're going to go all the way on these things or not."

"Well, I've thought of this. If my older brother's not there to make me come to therapy, I'm not coming."

I answered, "You'll have to decide what you're going to do about that. But your folks are still going to have to deal with the situation with you either way. You know, they need some help, too, or they wouldn't be here. Somebody who feels their family is that screwed up must feel their family needs some help."

"I don't think so."

"You think they're just fine the way they are?"

Mike countered with, "No. I think I should get out of the house as soon as possible."

The treatment of aggressive adolescents often begins with teenagers saying they want to live somewhere else. In most cases this proclamation is a guilt-tripping maneuver designed to keep parents off balance. Mr. and Mrs. Murphy had agreed that they would keep Mike home and do whatever it took to correct the problems. I repeated this to Mike and emphasized how committed to him they were. "They've said they're going to find ways at home to help you control your temper, and I'm going to help them control theirs, too—particularly your dad."

Mike responded with, "What are you going to do?"

I answered, "There might be a lot of things." My decision to answer Mike ambiguously piqued his interest. Mike sat up in his chair for the first time and responded with, "If he, like, got in a fight with my older brother, if he got in a fight with him, my older brother could probably take him down in 5 minutes or less."

Mike was warning me that his brother was the real power in the family. He was suggesting that there was risk of a dangerous confrontation between Jim and his father. The possibility of a fight between them worried Mike, but he kept a cold look in his eyes and talked as if he wanted his father hurt. I felt certain he was really worried his father might be hurt.

Mike continued, "And I would love to see that."

I changed the subject and probed at a nicer part of him, "I'm betting you still haven't decided you're really going to be a tough guy."

"What?" Mike asked, sounding surprised.

"I'm betting that you're just working on being a tough guy, and you're not all the way yet. Considering that you show interest in school—"

"I like school, and I like the school I'm at."

Sensing an opening, I said, "If you want to stay at your school, you're going to have to figure out how to get along with your parents."

Mike slumped back in his seat and answered, "I don't care. I'm not going to like them, no matter what."

"You don't believe they can change, but I may be able to help."

"Nothing you can do will help."

I continued, "What if I could work out some of the problems that bother you?"

"I don't care! I'm not going to like my family, no matter what," he answered angrily.

It was becoming clear to me that teaming up with Mike to help his family wasn't going to work. Hoping to salvage a small alliance, I pushed on to see if Mike might settle for our making the situation tolerable. "Would you be willing for us to work on making your home a place you could at least live with?"

Looking a bit confused and wrapping his arms around one knee, Mike said, "No! I don't know. I like our house and my school. But I don't like my parents."

Hopeful that I might be able to get an agreement, I pushed on: "Well, maybe that could be reason enough for me to have a chance to make the situation with your parents tolerable. Then you could stay in the same house, the same neighborhood—"

"It doesn't matter," he said with his head down, speaking slowly.

"You won't be able to stay at your school if you do anything as serious as you threaten."

Apparently, I'd challenged him too hard, because Mike suddenly got a more menacing look (much like the one he had at the beginning of the session) and said, "I know. I'll be sent to the juvenile center, and when I get out I'm going to kill my parents."

Although there was a moment when Mike seemed to be considering working with me, he contradicted any statement I made that was aimed at understanding his family's situation. Nevertheless, he did this in a way that gave me something concrete to work on. Later in the session Mike went on to tell me he'd kill me, too. This wasn't very convincing coming from a gangly prepubescent boy who had tears welling up in his eyes off and on throughout the interview. Mike made no threatening gestures toward me, and his threats had the quality of a kitten hissing at a dog. I couldn't figure out why previous therapists had believed him to be such a menace.

Although Mike refused to speak as if he were a nice guy, it was clear to me that he was worried about his family's welfare for some reason. Most importantly, I learned that he was a straight-A student at a difficult alternative school. (His teachers were all baffled by reports of his violent nature; they saw him as a delightful model student.)

It was important to end this critical first session in a way that gave the Murphys hope. When Mr. and Mrs. Murphy came back from the waiting room, I had to convince them that this therapy wouldn't be like the others, which had frightened and disempowered them with diagnoses, fearful predictions, and expert jargon. I had to take an immediate step that would begin to structure the situation; I had to define Mike's problems in terms that would put his parents in control and avoid further psychiatric involvement. I made a point of smiling at Mr. and Mrs. Murphy when I went to the waiting room to get them. Despite my best effort to act reassuring, they looked apprehensive as they sat down in my office with Mike. Even Mr. Murphy, who was a broad-shouldered, decisive man, looked worried. I immediately tried to put them at ease. "You know, you've got a nice son. He works at looking like a tough guy, but he doesn't really pull it off that well. You did something right with this one. In all likelihood, he's going to be okay, although he's got to make some decisions about how far he's willing to push things."

Mrs. Murphy seemed surprised and uncertain. "Okay," was all she said, though.

I continued, "Mike talks a lot about getting out of the house, but I don't think that's a good idea. I'd like the two of you to make a commitment to Mike today that the only thing that will get him out of your house is if he goes to jail. He's either a criminal or a kid in your family." By creating this dichotomy, that is, by challenging Mike to identify himself as a good guy or a criminal, I was walking a line between clarifying the options and goading Mike into criminal behavior. If I'd thought Mike was truly dangerous, this strategy would have been an error, for he would have felt compelled to defeat me by breaking the law and getting sent away. Not only did Mike's parents feel that he would never really hurt anyone, but I believed that he truly didn't want to be sent away. (A dichotomous position should also never be taken with a teenager who expresses a desire to commit suicide. If in doubt, the therapist should err on the side of caution and organize a high level of supervision and protection when either suicide or violence is threatened.)

Mrs. Murphy responded quickly to my request that they take a clear parental position, "He's a kid in our family. We've already told him that."

Mike muttered, "Unfortunately."

Mrs. Murphy continued with the strongest emotion I'd seen from her yet in the session: "He's not going back to the psychiatric hospital or anything like that."

Mr. Murphy wasn't talking yet. I was afraid this optimistic approach would alienate him. It seemed to me that he liked looking as if he was taking a hard line, which reminded me of Mike. To keep Mr. Murphy's interest, I emphasized the seriousness of Mike's threats to make this optimism look more forceful. I focused on Mike's behavior being bad rather than mad, so that his parents could begin thinking more clearly about their job of controlling inappropriate behavior. I knew that if I described Mike as mentally ill, his parents would feel frightened and hopeless and would have trouble taking action. On the other hand, if I presented his actions as serious misbehavior that could become criminal, his parents could continue to work on teaching him right from wrong. I began, "I don't think he needs psychiatric hospitalization. Mike's not mentally ill. If he does any of the violent acts he threatens, then he's a criminal."

Again, Mrs. Murphy jumped into the conversation first, turned toward Mike, and said, "Right. So you're stuck with us."

I was relieved when Mr. Murphy finally said, "I agree. I'll go along with that."

Thus, I was able to show Mike that his parents would respond to his threats as potential crimes rather than as a sign of mental illness. The 2-week period between this first session and the next was peaceful. The whole family—the parents and all three children—came to the next session.

Session 2: Beginning the Secret Weapon

My next task in the therapy was to continue containing and interrupting Mike's threats and frightening behaviors. To that end I suggested the approach now known as the secret weapon strategy, in which parents are asked to set a firm limit on the child's aggression and begin having their own secrets. I began the second session by identifying behavior both parents agreed would be way out of line. "Mr. and Mrs. Murphy, I would like you both to agree on a cutoff point that you, with one voice, could tell Mike is the point beyond which he may not go."

Again Mrs. Murphy started the discussion: "I'm willing to accept the verbal stuff, but I am not willing to accept him punching and breaking glasses and things like that."

As his mother spoke, Mike let his eyes wander around the room as if nothing were being said. Her halfhearted way of saying serious things just didn't penetrate his sorry show of bravado.

I clarified, "Okay, so your line would be when he becomes—"

"Physically aggressive, right," she finished for me.

To keep Mr. Murphy's interest I continued emphasizing the tough nature of this approach. "Now, I'm not saying you should tolerate swearing and disrespect. You'd probably do something very serious about it. How about you, Mr. Murphy?"

"I'll go along with her. I don't like it, but I'll go along. You know, I don't want to put up with the verbal abuse, either, but if she, I mean, most of it's directed at her. He won't give me verbal abuse because he knows I'll walk over and hit him."

Although he talked about hitting Mike, there wasn't any evidence of Mr. Murphy's ever having been violent. It would have been an error to jump on his statement as proof that a violent father was the cause of Mike's misbehavior. Instead, I listened for further concerns throughout the interview. I was beginning to think that Mike got his tendency toward bravado from his father. Because there was a possibility of abuse, it was important that I find indirect ways to clarify how often such instances of hitting Mike actually occurred. If I'd jumped to the conclusion that Mr. Murphy was abusive, a cycle of blaming the parents would have begun. As it turned out, I learned that Mr. Murphy hadn't been violent. If I had overreacted and had begun grilling Mr. Murphy about his behavior, I would have alienated one or both parents. Worse yet, Mrs. Murphy might have turned on Mr. Murphy and attacked him in response to my accusations.

If Mr. Murphy had in fact been violent with Mike, we would have needed to agree on a way of assuring that further violence wouldn't happen, but Mr. Murphy, like his younger son, only spoke *as if* he could be very dangerous. The more violent member of the family turned out to be Jim, Mike's 16-year-old brother. Jim, who was quite advanced in judo, disciplined Mike at his own discretion and without parental permission. Mr. and Mrs. Murphy saw Jim as a benevolent helper despite the level of violence he used on Mike. Mike's reference in the first therapy session to what would happen if Jim attacked his father made it clear that Jim's uncontrolled "helpfulness" was one of the threads interwoven in the fabric of this family's problem. As we set behavioral limits for Mike, I was thinking about how to stop Jim from attacking Mike and from disciplining him without permission. I commented, "You know, one of the things your folks said, Jim, is that they'd like to help you get out of the position where they need you to—"

"I don't mind," Jim interrupted.

"But they *are* your parents, and they have a sense of what's best for you."

It was already appearing that Jim liked the role of parental protector and that he might not give it up easily. Framed by his dark hair, Jim's deep brown eyes looked intent as he explained why he couldn't be spared as the family gladiator. "My mom can't climb stairs and my dad's incapacitated, so there's not much—"

Mr. Murphy, who had broken his ankle and was temporarily using a walker, interrupted Jim, saying, "Was I incapacitated the other night?"

Mrs. Murphy supported her husband, saying, "There's no way a 16-year-old should be in that position regularly."

Mr. Murphy echoed agreement. "We don't want you to have to act as a parent. We don't think it's fair to you."

Jim persisted. "Why? I don't mind."

Two adults weren't convincing enough, so I figured three might be able to make the point: "Your parents are right. It's not good for you to be correcting your brother. I'm glad you care enough about your family that you're willing to help, but the goal is to make it so that you won't be disciplining Mike."

When a sibling of a misbehaving adolescent is in a coalition with the parents, breaking up that alliance is a high priority. The sibling is allowing one parent to escape responsibilities by doing the job that parent should be doing. In addition, there's no reason why a troubled teenager should follow the directions of a brother or sister who's acting like a parent. The child who's acting like a parent may even be intentionally stirring up trouble to keep his or her place of authority in the family. In a single-parent family, this child may keep other adults from becoming involved by making it appear that the problem is being handled.

"Jim," I began, trying another approach, "you seem reluctant to give up the position of disciplinarian with Mike. I almost get the feeling that you like it. It gives you a position where you can really be helpful to your parents."

Jim finally gave me the ammunition I needed to challenge his motivation and insist that he stop. He answered, "In some ways I like to get back at him for what he does to me. That's another reason I like doing it."

I said to Jim, "I appreciate your honesty." I really meant that I appreciated this admission, which I would later use to stop him from punishing Mike. Mike's parents were agreeing with me, but without much conviction or passion. Therefore, I continued to dramatize the dangerousness of Mike's behavior, by using emotional language, until the parents' affect reflected more conviction: "We need to help Mike stop making statements that could get him killed if he says them to the wrong person. What I'd like you to do is stop his behavior before something terrible happens. Then you've got the luxury of taking your time and working out the other problems like swearing."

Mrs. Murphy answered, "Okay."

Again her answer was spoken in a rather meek voice and wasn't echoed by her husband, so I continued dramatizing the situation, trying to draw him in. Mr. Murphy was very logical so I appealed to his logical sense of the need for consequences for Mike: "Most of what Mike says he'll do, as we've talked about before, isn't crazy, it's criminal. In fact, in the eyes of the law, going out and telling somebody you're going to kill them is assault. I don't know if you know that."

Mr. Murphy immediately showed some interest and indicated that he'd just then begun listening to me: "Say that again?"

I repeated, "If you go out on the streets and tell somebody you're going to kill them, that's assault."

Still interested, Mr. Murphy said, "Oh, I didn't know that."

Because this tack seemed to be generating some enthusiasm, I elaborated: "Yes. Assault and battery is if you physically do something to someone."

Mr. Murphy completed the thought with, "Assault is just verbally saying, 'I'm going to kill you.' "

For the first time this session, both Mr. and Mrs. Murphy began talking with some animation. Mike was shifting around in his seat and seemed a little nervous. He was looking back and forth from one parent to the other as if realizing that they were finally seeing his behavior as criminal rather than crazy; he seemed surprised that they might both agree on that view. Now that I had their attention and had brought about a shift in their affect, I returned to the secret weapon strategy and my attempt to get the Murphys to agree on limits to Mike's behavior that would keep him from acting dangerously. "There has to be a plan in place so we know Mike's behavior isn't going to go beyond the point of threats," I said. "Mike has to understand where the cutoff point is. He has to know these limits come from both of you as a team and no one else." With Mike still looking nervous, I tried to include him in the conversation. The fact that he hadn't interrupted showed me he really wanted his parents to agree on something. "So you've heard today what your mom and dad said about what the cutoff point is. Right, Mike?"

Rather halfheartedly, he tried to be his usual arrogant self and answered, "No, I don't listen. They're stupid, just like you."

Keeping to the task at hand I answered, "Okay, he heard it. Between now and the next time we get together, I'd like the two of you to have a talk when none of the other kids are around. We don't want Jim to be any more in the middle of things than he has to be."

It is an old Ericksonian technique to begin telling someone what you want them to do and then wander off onto another thought. I almost assigned Mr. and Mrs. Murphy some homework, but then I moved to finishing the job of stopping Jim's violence toward Mike. I figured that by the time I finally gave the parents their task, they would be that much more inclined to do it. I turned to Jim and said, "You know, I appreciate your willingness to be there for physical support if it's needed, but we want to make that as little as possible."

Jim answered, "Right now it would be difficult for me not to."

Unconvinced, I continued, "Uh-huh. Well, I'm going to ask you to do something with us, Jim. I'm going to ask you not to do anything physical toward Mike unless your parents request it of you."

He answered, "Okay."

"Good, that's going to keep you from getting in trouble."

Jim said, "I don't usually get in trouble, anyways."

Mike echoed, "He never gets caught for doing anything."

I made the point by saying, "Now you will." As if there hadn't been any discussion in between, I then picked up where I had left off with Mr. and Mrs. Murphy: "And, what I'd like you to do is, I'd like you both to come up with something that's going to happen to Mike that'll be worse than having to control himself if he ever crosses that line again into dangerous behavior. But I want you to come up with something so insidious—"

I knew I was making progress when Mr. Murphy said with a mischievous look, "Just one thing?"

"Just one thing," I agreed.

I seemed to have managed a balance between the parents' different styles. Mr. Murphy saw that serious problems were going to be addressed with serious consequences. Mrs. Murphy saw that only serious infractions were going to be handled that sternly. The limitations on harsh consequences helped relieve Mrs. Murphy's concern that one of her children and her husband were going to wind up in a physical fight and hurt each other.

However, I was still nervous about that comment Mr. Murphy had made earlier about hitting Mike if he talked back. It was time to handle that concern within the context of the secret weapon strategy. Metaphorically, we were discussing Mike's behavior and the threat of a possible physical battle between Mr. Murphy and Jim in the future. "Frankly, the most insidious things parents can do almost never have to do with anything physical being required. We just wind up in power struggles with teenagers who are getting bigger than us. So I think you need to come up with something *really* insidious. There'll be no negotiation on what happens when that line gets crossed. It's got to be harder on him than the effort it would take for Mike to control himself to that point."

Mike again tried to divert the discussion with a threat and said, "I should try that." He was referring to crossing the line of dangerousness his parents had defined for him during the session.

To end the discussion I said to Mike, "You can try acting dangerously. But the outside world generally isn't as understanding as your parents about being abused. And they've decided to stop being so understanding."

Leaning forward with a mischievous grin, Mr. Murphy chimed in, "How about that big guy Jeff on the bus? Why don't you go try and offend him?"

Mike answered, "Okay, I will. He won't do anything."

If therapy is to be successful, the therapist must show the parents that they can get back in control of their children. The best sign of this renewed control is when parents are no longer reacting to their child's provocation and are, in fact, doing a bit of playful provoking themselves. At this point in the therapy, Mr. and Mrs. Murphy were taking positions with Mike that were throwing him off balance and making him think about how he was going to respond. Mr. and Mrs. Murphy seemed quite unified. I was pleased to see that Mrs. Murphy had a small smile on her face as she watched the conversation between her husband and son; she was looking amused rather than fearful. I kept moving forward with the discussion of the strategy without leaving pauses in the conversation that might encourage interruptions or diversions: "So, what's going to happen is, he's going to say and do things that make you think he's crossed that line. You should talk together about examples of what might constitute crossing that line. Because when you're talking about doing something this big, you've got to make sure that the line was crossed."

Session 3: The Response

Mr. and Mrs. Murphy brought all three children to the third session. Everyone seemed to walk with a lighter step as they came into the room and sat down. Instead of sitting on opposite sides of the room as they had in the first session, Mr. and Mrs. Murphy sat beside each other with the children arrayed on both sides of them. I saw this as evidence that their sense of unity as a couple had improved. Mrs. Murphy seemed transformed. Smiling and sitting more erect, she looked cheerful and relaxed. Both parents agreed that Mike had stopped all aggression and threats of violence.

Although I still had to finish the secret weapon strategy, I had to address another issue. I was afraid the improvement in Mike might not last if the cause for his painful feelings was not addressed. I had hypothesized that his threats of violence and murder were messages about his family that had previously been ignored. Mike's message told me that family members hadn't recovered from the deaths of the people they loved. As long as the family was preoccupied with Mike, they avoided lapsing into depression and grief over their losses. I believed that Mike's threats of violence were occurring simultaneously with family members' deep feelings about death and loss. Both grandmothers had died in the recent past, and Mrs. Murphy often mentioned how those grandparents would have felt about Mike's behavior. By presenting Mike as the symptom bearer, the family was telling me that their grief would be discussed through him. In keeping with their unspoken request to use Mike as an avenue for discussing loss, I talked about how the deaths of his grandparents had affected Mike, but I avoided connecting Mike's grief to the grief the rest of the family was going through: "It seems like a lot of Mike's behavior has gotten worse since his grandma died. I understand that you guys were real close to your grandma, too."

Jim said, "I don't remember."

Mrs. Murphy commented, "Yeah, she was over a lot. Jim, what do you mean, you don't remember? She baby-sat a lot. I'd say things seemed to be worse after Grandma died as far as more misbehaving, particularly by Mike and probably with Jim."

Jim launched into a long discussion about how the death of his grandmother hadn't affected him. He argued that he simply put the deaths out of his mind and claimed that solved the problem. I thought he was speaking for the whole family, so I answered him for the whole family: "Unfortunately, we're all ruled by certain laws of nature. Death is the one experience that overshadows everything, no matter how rationally we try to think about it."

I had entered a realm close to Mrs. Murphy's heart. She spoke in a softer, warmer voice saying, "Well, this was so sudden, you know. They expected their grandpa's death because he'd been very ill, and it was almost like a blessing when he died. But with their grandma, they had just seen her, they'd talked to her the night before, and then she was gone the next morning. And they happened to be off from school, so they were with me when I drove down to her house and found her. She was 71."

Jim corrected, "No, she was 76."

Mr. Murphy said, "Yeah, I thought she was older."

Jim showed us that he remembered details about his grandmother very well. I moved the conversation back to the family's interaction with her. "Did you guys stay over at her house when you were younger?"

Jim volunteered, "A lot, when we were younger, yeah."

Mr. Murphy added, "And up until very close to the end Jim and Mike still went over and would stay overnight. Grandma had these Saturday things; you know, she gave them everything."

"They went Friday night and came home Sunday afternoon," said Mrs. Murphy.

Mr. Murphy continued, "Yeah, it was a big production thing that Grandma got a kick out of, and so did the boys. We thought she spoiled them but Grandma seemed to enjoy it so I didn't complain too much."

Smiling, Mrs. Murphy remembered, "Yeah, we had a usual joke. They'd go to Grandma's for the weekend, and when we picked them up Sunday afternoon, we'd shake them and say, 'Welcome back to reality.'"

Even Mike surprised himself and got caught laughing. I was moved by the warmth being expressed by this group of apparently cold, depressed people. Because of this dramatic shift in the family's emotions, I was also reassured that we were discussing the subject that was troubling Mike and his family.

When he saw Mike laughing, Mr. Murphy tried to bring him into the conversation. "You used to enjoy going over to Grandma's."

"Yeah."

"And I know you were probably as helpful as any of the three," Mr. Murphy continued.

With an unconvincing sneer Mike said, "That's because she would let us do absolutely anything." Mike was sitting forward in his seat now, and there was more color in his face. He was still hesitant to let himself be seen as a good guy, so he resisted any statement that implied niceness on his part.

Mr. Murphy kept trying to draw Mike out. "Yeah, but you cleaned up around the house for her a couple of times. I know you did."

Mike retorted, "Yeah, and then all the stuff I found I either took apart or broke."

With a grin Mrs. Murphy added, "You'd go over with one suitcase, and come home with one suitcase and two bags full."

"Yeah, tape recorders I'd find, and I'd take them apart," Mike laughed. "Just ask Bonnie. She remembers."

Bonnie didn't really look as if she wanted to get into the conversation yet, so I let her be for a while longer. Keeping to the subject of the kindness of grandmothers, I said, "Grandmas are real patient. I remember my grandma. I'd go over there and I knew that anything I came across in the house that I admired, she'd give it to me."

Mrs. Murphy laughed, "Yeah."

I'd encouraged a discussion that had the children talking about their time with their grandmother. There was a new feeling in the room, one that made it possible for me to discuss how everyone was dealing with the loss. Neither Mr. nor Mrs. Murphy had referred to the boys' grandmother as Mrs. Murphy's mother, so I concluded that doing so would cause Mrs. Murphy so much pain that her newly acquired positive mood might shatter. Since I was concerned about her depression over the loss of her mother, I moved slowly and abstractly into a discussion of loss. "You know, it's a shame, really, that it happens like that sometimes after someone dies. People deal with it the same way you do, Jim. They not only push the death out of their minds, they push the memory of what they had together out of their minds, too."

Jim defended himself, saying, "That's one of the bad things about it but it works for me so that's what I do."

As I pursued the subject of how people avoid dealing with loss, I equalized the brothers, putting Jim and Mike on the same level. I presented both brothers as having trouble recovering from the death of their grandmother. I assumed that the trouble the children were having revealed something about the family's problematic style for dealing with loss. Everyone felt more comfortable dealing with Mike's allusions to death and murder than with the grief that was hovering and waiting to be experienced. I kept the focus on Mike so that the defenses of the other family members wouldn't rise up and interrupt what I was saying: "I think Mike handles death by avoiding it, too. He does it with a sense of humor or by cranking things up so the whole subject changes. I don't think I'm of the same religion you are, but I was raised Jewish. Jews have one central belief—that if someone is forgotten, then they're really dead. Bonnie, what do you remember about your grandma?"

Bonnie sheepishly answered, "Not much. Well, she always would take me to the store. Every time I go there, she'd either take me to the store and take me out to a movie or take me miniature golfing."

Mrs. Murphy empathized, "Yeah, that was fun, miniature golfing."

Bonnie chuckled, "Yeah."

Mrs. Murphy had to prompt Bonnie a lot to get an answer, and Bonnie still tried to sound disinterested. I used this opportunity to again make the point that the family hadn't adequately dealt with the deaths. "We're talking about her grandma, and Bonnie's sort of saying, 'When are we going home? Can we stop this conversation?'"

I'd pointed out that all three children were using troubled methods for dealing with the loss of a beloved grandparent. Although I assumed that Mr. and Mrs. Murphy were also mishandling the death, I kept the focus on the children. There was enough evidence to justify my issuing a directive for helping the children deal with the loss, a directive for a ritual that would include and help the whole family. Looking at Mr. and Mrs. Murphy, I said, "Let me ask you to do something else. I'd like to ask you to pick a tabletop or counter in a room everybody's going to be going through and make a memorial to their grandmother. Photographs, belongings, things that are going to—"

Before I could finish, Mr. Murphy showed me that his wife was the family member most upset over the loss by turning to her and asking, "Can you handle that personally?" Mrs. Murphy nodded her agreement. Mr. Murphy suggested, "We've got pictures."

Mrs. Murphy said, "There are pictures on the wall."

He said, "We'll put the pictures over on the counter plus we'll go through a couple of scrapbooks."

Keeping the obvious enthusiasm going, I suggested, "Maybe you can help the kids pick some of the things they were given by their grandmother to put on the memorial."

"Yeah, they have several things," agreed Mrs. Murphy.

Mr. Murphy turned to Mike and asked, "You have a couple of those keys, don't you?"

Mike started to ask, "What kind of—" but got cut off by a jumble of voices talking at the same time.

Mrs. Murphy said, "Bonnie, you have the pictures that were on your wall and on your bookcase. My mom painted quite a bit." The last comment was directed at me.

Mike showed another sign of humor by adding, "I got her TV."

Mrs. Murphy used her hands to show the dimensions of a large television set, chuckled, and said, "I don't know about the TV."

The animated, cheerful family in my office didn't bear much resemblance to the one that came for therapy 2 weeks earlier. When I see this kind of incredible affective shift, I usually conclude that I've struck gold. As the session wound down, I ended the planning for the memorial by saying, "I don't really know about formal afterlife, but I believe that if people do live on, it's through the people who love them."

The directive approach to therapy is unique in that we therapists feel free to keep the troubled adolescent as the focus of therapy—as opposed to convincing parents that they have a family problem. A therapist who directs statements at the troubled adolescent can say things he or she wants the parents or siblings to hear. Because other family members don't realize that they're being addressed, they relax and accept the message more readily than if the therapist tries to make a difficult point directly. I used this approach as I discussed death and grief with the Murphy children; that is, I spoke as if they alone were having trouble recovering from the loss of their grandmother.

Session 4: Arming the Secret Weapon

The whole family arrived for the fourth session. I met with Mr. and Mrs. Murphy first to discuss their choice of the secret weapon. They insisted on two consequences because their list had both very serious and not so serious misbehaviors on it. The milder secret weapon was more like an ordinary consequence for misbehavior, but I supported their choice because they were so unified about it. I learned at this session that Mike had studied to be a clown and had even gone to Clown College of the Ringling Bros. and Barnum & Bailey Circus. He belonged to a unicycle club and practiced riding a lot. He rode with a unicycle brigade in at least one parade every month. His parents' first secret weapon was to take his unicycle and lock it in a friend's garage for a month. I was surprised that they considered this extreme, and it helped me understand how hesitant they'd been in the past to do anything really powerful.

The second secret weapon for serious infractions, unlike the first intervention, was a true atom bomb. If Mike violated the guidelines for dangerousness, his parents intended to show school personnel a copy of a videotape from a therapy session in which Mike had behaved badly, threatening murder, and sworn at adults. Mike was a very good student and well liked by teachers. He felt supported in his anger at his parents by school personnel, who thought he was wonderful. The school faculty often acted as if they thought there were something wrong with Mr. and Mrs. Murphy because they claimed that Mike had behavioral problems at home. With the videotape the Murphys would be able to show school personnel the kind of behavior Mike displayed within the family.

On the surface, showing the videotape to the school looked like a cruel act that would handicap the one area of Mike's life in which he felt successful. Concern over depriving their child of a positive experience is a reason parents often give for not taking away sports or other beloved activities. I felt comfortable supporting the Murphys' choice because I didn't think we had much to lose. Mike wouldn't get to stay at that school if he continued to act crazy and were placed in residential treatment or the juvenile detention facility. He'd already spent 2 weeks in a psychiatric hospital away from school.

After my meeting with Mr. and Mrs. Murphy, I then met with the whole family. I began moving right ahead with the completion of the strategy, that is, with the procedure by which the secret weapon is armed. To Mr. and Mrs. Murphy I said, "To recap, you're helping Mike keep his behavior within a reasonable range. I asked the two of you to go home and decide on something you'll do that would be worse than Mike having to control himself. (*to Mike*) Being the creative folks your parents are, they thought of two."

I could really see the change when Mrs. Murphy spoke first and said, "Yeah, we have two doozies."

True to form, Mike asked, "Will you tell them to me?"

Mrs. Murphy answered, "Uh-uh."

I reinforced her position saying, "You only get to find out one way." Bonnie nervously walked across the room, put down a piece of paper, and walked back to her seat. "That's something for your parents to know and, hopefully, for nobody to ever find out. Maybe when you get married or graduate from college, they'll tell you as part of your gift."

Mike immediately interrupted and pointed at his parents, threatening, "When I graduate college, they won't be alive."

Unable to get information he wanted, Mike resorted to threatening to murder his parents. The test at this point in the therapy was whether Mr. and Mrs. Murphy would respond with terror and lose their focus or refuse to act frightened and continue to withhold the information from Mike. I began challenging Mike's threat in a slightly playful way. I hoped his parents would follow my lead and keep their balance. The way I began—by discussing how people die, which tied in with our previous discussion about his grandmother—also gave Mike an opportunity to back out of the position he was taking.

"Really?" I said. "Do you really think people die that easily?"

"No. I'm going to kill them," Mike said matter-of-factly. By making his threat explicit, Mike had committed himself to testing whether there would be a consequence.

"Oh, I see," I said, turning to Mr. and Mrs. Murphy. "I think you're going to have to do one of those two things. He just threatened murder. Do the first one tonight."

Mike smiled and said, "I get to find out what one of them is."

"Yep," I agreed.

Mr. Murphy surprised me by saying, "I think he's just pulling our chain, frankly. I don't think he's threatening us."

I just said, "Don't you?"

I didn't know if Mr. Murphy was backing down from taking action, which would ruin the intervention, or if he was saying that he and his wife no longer found Mike's threats convincing and that they would no longer take them seriously. I waited and crossed my fingers.

Mr. Murphy turned to his wife, again a good sign, and asked, "Do you think he's threatening us?"

Without hesitation she answered, "I don't think he is."

Mr. Murphy gestured toward the cast on his leg and ratified their agreement by saying, "Yeah. I'll give you a prime example. I went and spanked him one night. He says, 'I'm going to kick you and push you down the stairs.' I turned around and put my back to him. I didn't look at him, and I said, 'Go ahead.' I mean, I thought the kid was mad enough that he might actually do it, but he didn't."

Mrs. Murphy joined in, saying, "I agree. Those are words. That's not action."

I was relieved that Mr. and Mrs. Murphy seemed to be taking a strong position rather than a weak one. In support of them I emphasized, "So he'd have to be more convincing if you were to consider it a violation of the cutoff point. You're saying that he wasn't even convincing."

Mrs. Murphy said, "No."

"Not when he's sitting there smiling," agreed Mr. Murphy.

Mike didn't make any further threats after that session. The Murphys and I met for eight more sessions and worked out contracts for age-appropriate rights and responsibilities for each child. I intervened in minor behavior problems and even negotiated some financial agreements between Mr. and Mrs. Murphy that they'd asked for help with. The Murphys reported that Mike was behaving like the boy they'd known before he started making threats but that he still tended to be a bit surly at times.

The following excerpt from the ninth therapy session characterizes the change in Mike's manner and in the interactions between family members. (Mr. Murphy had to work the day of this particular session but had been attending sessions regularly.)

"Did you guys go to the circus this year?" I began.

Mrs. Murphy was smiling when she said, "We were in row three, where they all come out. It was real nice."

Still being a bit disagreeable, Mike said, "It was dumb. The main attraction was some guy wrestling a drugged alligator." He had a smirk on his face as he spoke.

I laughed, "A drugged alligator? I saw some previews of that on TV. It wasn't that impressive, huh?"

He said, "It was drugged. It could barely take two steps."

Mrs. Murphy agreed, "Well, the tank was right in front of us. You know, he gets in and wrestles this thing."

Mike completed the thought: "The alligator is trying to get to the top for air and he jumps in and pulls his neck back and forth out of the water."

Mrs. Murphy was laughing now. "It was bad. But the clowns were real good, and that's what we went for."

"Oh, yeah. That would be more interesting for you, wouldn't it, Mike?" I asked.

"I love the clowns," Mike said. He had been holding some juggling balls since the beginning of the session.

Taking the cue, I motioned toward the balls and asked, "Will you show me some things?"

Mike stood up and started doing some impressive juggling, which made him move around the room. His mother looked proud. I was tickled. "Did you teach yourself or did somebody teach you?"

"I taught myself."

It was at that session that I began describing Mike as the family entertainer, as the one with a dramatic and theatrical flair. I likened him to the entertainment director on a cruise ship. Treatment ended after 11 sessions. Mr. and Mrs. Murphy came back for a few sessions to get a bit of advice over the next 4 years, and I got follow-up information about the children at those times. I learned that Mike had completed his education at the private school and had entered public high school, as intended. He did reasonably well throughout high school, but his parents had to give him some greater structure when his grades dropped to B's and C's during his junior year. He also got quite a few speeding tickets after he got his driver's license. Jim may have set the world's record for the number of universities and majors a student can go through while keeping an almost straight-A average at all of them. As of 4 years after the therapy, there hadn't been a recurrence of violent or aggressive behavior by any of the children. Bonnie stayed quietly in the background and continued doing fine. Mr. and Mrs. Murphy, though asking for marital advice at times, continued to be pleased with their marriage.

CONCLUSION

The course of therapy with abusive adolescents is determined by the presence or absence of a diagnosis. Therapists must make a choice between normalizing the lives of adolescents in distress or exacerbating everyone's fears with hospitalizations and medication. The act of thinking in diagnostic labels directs therapists toward greater assumptions of disturbance. As discussed in the preceding chapters, thinking in terms of steps back toward normality provides a commonsense guide to improvement.

References

Andersen, T. *The reflecting team*. New York: Norton, 1991.

Andersen, T. See and hear, and be seen and heard. In *The new language of change* (S. Friedman, ed.). New York: Guilford Press, 1993.

Association for Humanistic Psychology. *The meaning of humanistic psychology*. San Francisco: Author, 1987.

Berg, I. K., & de Shazer, S. Making numbers talk: Language in therapy. In *The new language of change* (S. Friedman, ed.). New York: Guilford Press, 1993.

Bergman, J. *Fishing for barracuda*. New York: Norton, 1985.

Boswell, R. *Mystery ride*. New York: Knopf, 1992.

Deighton, J., & McPeek, P. Group treatment: Adult victims of childhood sexual abuse. *Social Casework*, 1985.

de Shazer, S. *Keys to solutions in brief therapy*. New York: Norton, 1985.

Guest, J. *Ordinary people*. New York: Viking, 1976.

Gurman, A. S., & Kniskern, D. P. Family therapy research: Knowns and unknowns. In *Handbook of family therapy* (A. S. Gurman & D. P. Kniskern, eds.). New York: Brunner/Mazel, 1991.

Haley, J. *Strategies of psychotherapy*. New York: Grune & Stratton, 1964.

Haley, J. *Problem solving therapy*. San Francisco: Jossey-Bass, 1976.

Haley, J. *Leaving home*. New York: McGraw-Hill, 1980.

Hoff, B. *The tao of Pooh*. New York: Penguin Books, 1982.

Lamont, C. *The philosophy of humanism*. New York: Continuum, 1990.

Lao Tsu. *The tao te ching* (trans. by G.-F. Feng & J. English; Intro. by J. Needleman). New York: Vintage Books, 1989.

Lawson, G., & Lawson, A. *Adolescent substance abuse*. Gaithersberg, MD: Aspen, 1992.

Madanes, C. *Strategic family therapy*. San Francisco: Jossey-Bass, 1981.

Madanes, C. *Behind the one-way mirror*. San Francisco: Jossey-Bass, 1984.

Madanes, C. *Sex, love, and violence*. New York: Norton, 1990.

Minuchin, S. *Families and family therapy*. Cambridge, MA: Harvard University Press, 1974.

Minuchin, S., & Fishman, H. C. *Family therapy techniques*. Cambridge, MA: Harvard University Press, 1981.

National Institute on Drug Abuse and University of Michigan Institute for Social

Research. *Drug use among American high school seniors, college students, and young adults 1975–1990*. Rockville, MD: Author, 1991.

Nichols, M. P. The therapist as authority figure. *Family Process, 32,* 163–165, 1993.

O'Hanlon, W., & Weiner-Davis, M. *In search of solutions: A new direction in psychotherapy*. New York: Norton, 1989.

Palazzoli, M. S., Cirillo, S., Selvini, M., & Sorrentino, A. *Family games*. New York: Norton, 1989.

Price, J. A. A strategic approach to accessing the families of adolescents. *Journal of Strategic and Systemic Therapies, 6*(1), 67–72, 1987.

Price, J. A. How to stabilize families. *Journal of Strategic and Systemic Therapies, 7*(4), 24–27, 1988.

Saposnek, D. Aikido: A model for brief strategic therapy. *Family Process, 19,* 227–238, 1980.

U.S. Department of Health and Human Services. *Guideline for the treatment of alcohol and other drug abusing adolescents*. Rockville, MD: Author, 1993.

Whitaker, C. *Midnight musings of a family therapist*. New York: Norton, 1989.

Index